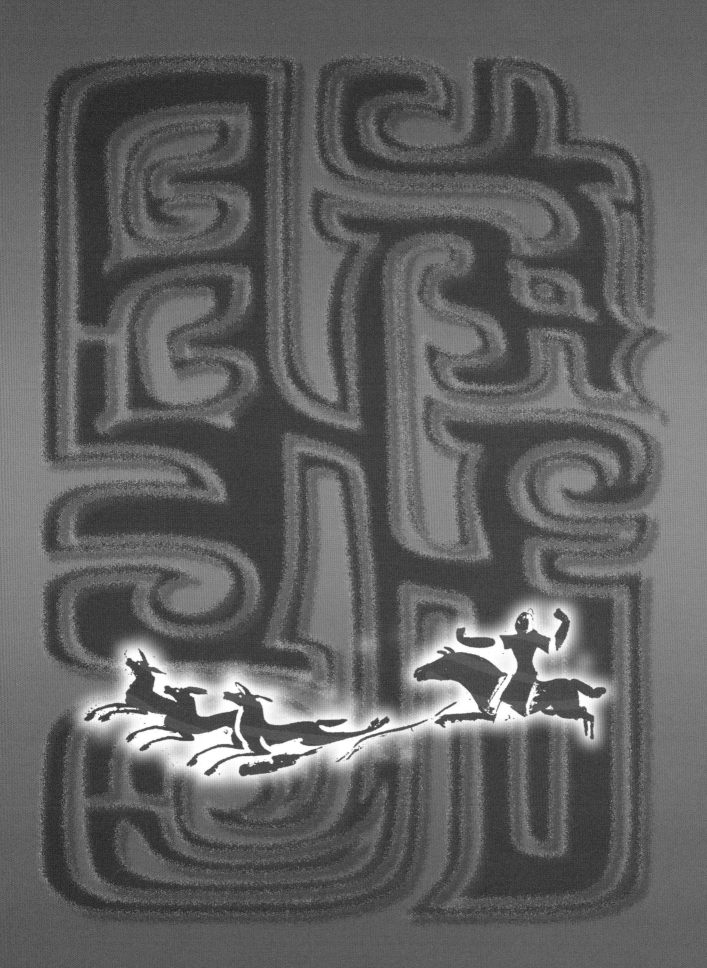

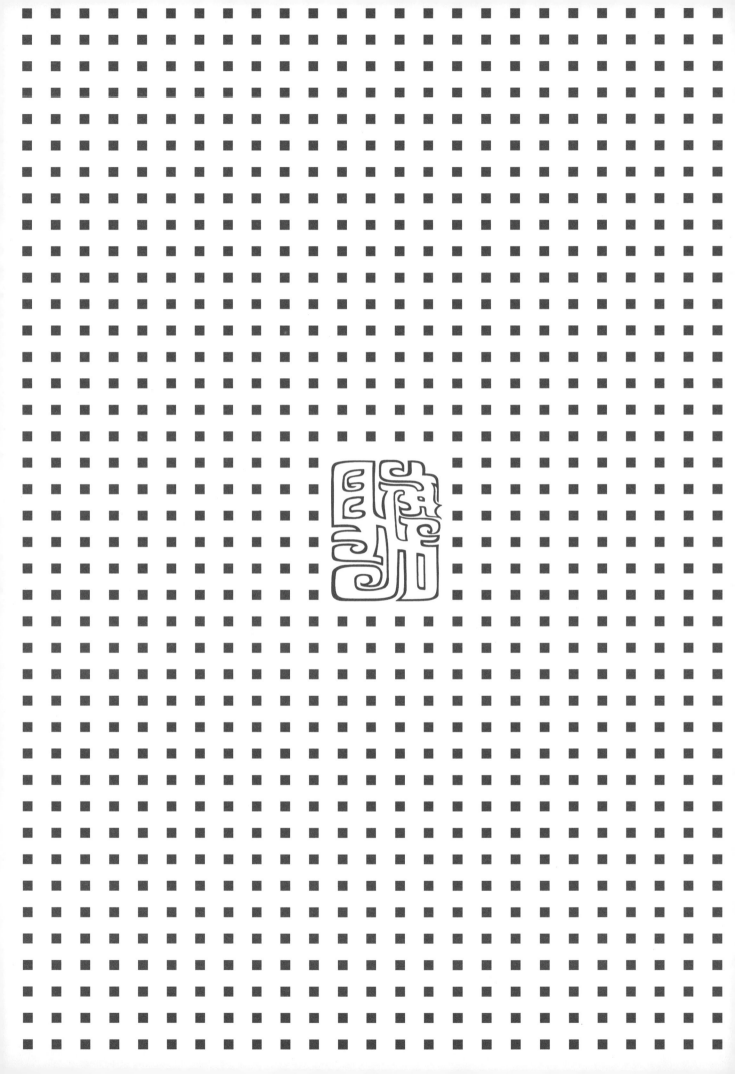

国家出版基金项目
NATIONAL PUBLICATION FOUNDATION

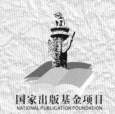

中华医药卫生

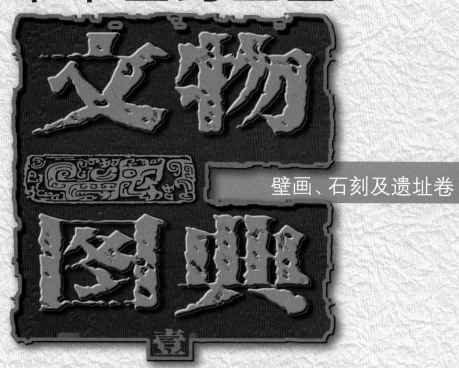

壁画、石刻及遗址卷

主　编　李经纬　梁　峻　刘学春
总主译　白永权
主　译　赵永生

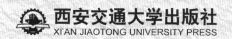

西安交通大学出版社
XI'AN JIAOTONG UNIVERSITY PRESS

图书在版编目 (CIP) 数据

中华医药卫生文物图典 . 1. 壁画、石刻及遗址卷 / 李经纬，

梁峻，刘学春主编 . — 西安：西安交通大学出版社，2016.12

ISBN 978-7-5605-7014-3

Ⅰ . ①中… Ⅱ . ①李… ②梁… ③刘… Ⅲ . ①中国医药学—

壁画—中国—古代 - 图录②中国医药学—石刻—中国—古

代—图录③中国医药学—文化遗址—中国—图录 Ⅳ . ① R-092 ② K870.2

中国版本图书馆 CIP 数据核字（2015）第 013594 号

书　　名　中华医药卫生文物图典（一）壁画、石刻及遗址卷

主　　编　李经纬　梁　峻　刘学春

责任编辑　赵文娟

出版发行　西安交通大学出版社

　　　　　（西安市兴庆南路 10 号　邮政编码 710049）

网　　址　http://www.xjtupress.com

电　　话　（029）82668805　82668502（医学分社）

　　　　　（029）82668315（总编办）

传　　真　（029）82668280

印　　刷　中煤地西安地图制印有限公司

开　　本　889mm×1194mm　1/16　印张 21.25　字数　346 千字

版次印次　2017 年 12 月第 1 版　2017 年 12 月第 1 次印刷

书　　号　ISBN 978-7-5605-7014-3

定　　价　680.00 元

读者购书、书店添货、如发现印装质量问题，请通过以下方式联系、调换。

订购热线：（029）82665248　（029）82665249

投稿热线：（029）82668805　（029）82668502

读者信箱：medpress@126.com

铭记感受历史

自信自重自强

书贺

中华医药卫生文物图典问世

陈可冀 谨题

二○一七年六月

陈可冀　中国科学院院士、国医大师

精修醫藥衛生文物

圖典功著當代

深究岐黃學術思想

淵源惠澤千秋

中華醫藥衛生文物圖典出版誌慶

丁酉孟秋 孫光榮 敬題於北京

孫光荣　国医大师

中華醫藥衛生文物圖典出版

彰顯中醫藥
文化精神

體現中醫藥
歷史價值

歲次丁酉夏　王琦

王琦　国医大师

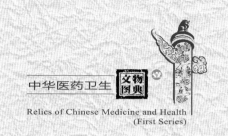

Relics of Chinese Medicine and Health
(First Series)

中华医药卫生文物图典（一）
丛书编撰委员会

主　编　李经纬　梁　峻　刘学春

副主编　廖　果　吴鸿洲　康兴军　和中浚　刘小斌　杨金生

　　　　郑怀林　徐江雁　白建疆　黄　煌

编　委　李洪晓　梁永宣　王强虎　董树平　马　健　王　霞

　　　　张雅宗　朱德明　包哈申　张建青　郑　蓉　庄乾竹

　　　　李宏红　刘哲峰　王宏才　陈润东

总主译　白永权

主　译　陈向京　聂文信　范晓晖　温　睿　赵永生　杜彦龙

　　　　吉　乐　李小棉　郭　梦　陈　曦

副主译（按姓氏音序排列）

　　　　董艳云　姜雨孜　李建西　刘　慧　马　健　任宝磊

　　　　任　萌　任　莹　王　颇　习通源　谢皖吉　徐素云

　　　　许崇钰　许　梅　詹菊红　赵　菲　邹郝晶

译　者（按姓氏音序排列）

迟征宇　邓　甜　付一豪　高　琛　高　媛　郭　宁

韩　蕾　何宗昌　胡勇强　黄　鋆　蒋新蕾　康晓薇

李静波　刘雅恬　刘妍萌　鲁显生　马　月　牛笑语

唐云鹏　唐臻娜　田　多　铁红玲　佟健一　王　晨

王　丹　王　栋　王　丽　王　媛　王慧敏　王梦杰

王仙先　吴耀均　席　慧　肖国强　许子洋　闫红贤

杨姣姣　姚　晔　张　阳　张　鋆　张继飞　张梦原

张晓谦　赵　欣　赵亚力　郑　青　郑艳华　朱江嵩

朱瑛培

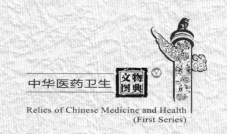

Relics of Chinese Medicine and Health
(First Series)

本册编撰委员会

主　编　李经纬　梁　峻　刘学春

副主编　廖　果　吴鸿洲　康兴军　和中浚　刘小斌　杨金生
　　　　　郑怀林　徐江雁　白建疆　黄　煌

编　委　李洪晓　梁永宣　王强虎　董树平　马　健　王　霞
　　　　　张雅宗　朱德明　包哈申　张建青　郑　蓉　庄乾竹
　　　　　李宏红　刘哲峰　王宏才　陈润东

总主译　白永权

主　译　赵永生

副主译　徐素云

译　者　许崇钰　铁红玲　邓　甜

丛书策划委员会

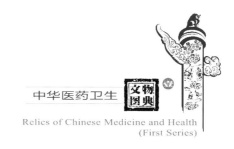

中华医药卫生 文物图典

Relics of Chinese Medicine and Health
(First Series)

序　言

　　探索天、地、人运动变化规律以及"气化物生"过程的相互关系，是人类永恒的课题。宇宙不可逆，地球不可逆，人生不可逆业已成为共识。天地造化形成自然，人类活动构成文化。文物既是文化的载体，又是物化的历史，还是文明的见证。

　　追求健康长寿是人类共同的夙愿。中华民族之所以繁衍昌盛，健康文化起了巨大的推动作用。由于古人谋求生存发展、应对环境变化产生的智慧，大多反映在以医药卫生为核心的健康文化之中，所以，习总书记说："中医药学是中国古代科学的瑰宝，也是打开中华文明宝库的钥匙"。

　　秉持文化大发展、大繁荣理念，中国中医科学院李经纬、梁峻等为负责人的科研团队在完成科技部"国家重点医药卫生文物收集调研和保护"课题获 2005 年度中华中医药学会科技二等奖基础上，又资鉴"夏商周断代工程""中华文明探源工程"等相关考古成果，用有重要价值的新出土文物置换原拍摄质量较差的文物，适当补充民族医药文物，共精选收载 5000 余件。经西安交通大学出版社申报，《中华医药卫生文物图典（一）》（以下简称《图典》）于 2013 年获得了国家出版基金的资助，并经专业翻译团队翻译，使《图典》得以面世。

　　文物承载的信息多元丰富，发掘解读其中蕴藏的智慧并非易事。医药卫生文物更具有特殊性，除文物的一般属性外，还承载着传统医学发展史迹与促进健康的信息。运用历史唯物主义观察发掘文物信息，善于从生活文物中领悟卫生信息，才能准确解读其功能，也才能诠释其在民生健康中的历史作用，收到以古鉴今之效果。"历史是现实的根源"，任何一个民族都不能割断历史，史料都包含在文化中。"文化是民族的血脉，是人民的精神家园"，文化繁荣才能实现中华民族的伟大复兴。值本《图典》付梓之际，用"梳理文化之脉，必获健康之果"作为序言并和作者、读者共勉！

中央文史研究馆馆员
中国工程院院士　　王永炎
丁酉年仲夏

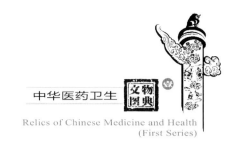

中华医药卫生 文物图典

Relics of Chinese Medicine and Health
(First Series)

前　言

　　文化是相对自然的概念，是考古界常用词汇。文物是文化的重要组成部分，既是文明的物证，又是物化的历史。狭义医药卫生文物是疾病防治模式语境下的解读，而广义医药卫生文物则是躯体、心态、环境适应三维健康模式下的诠释。中华民族是 56 个民族组成的多元一体大家庭，中华医药卫生文物当然包括各民族的健康文化遗存。

　　天地造化如造山、板块漂移、气候变迁、生物起源进化等形成自然。气化物生莫贵于人，即整个生物进化的最高成果是人类自身。广义而言，人类生存思维留下的痕迹即物质财富和精神财富总和构成文化，其一般的物化形式是视觉感知的文物、文献、胜迹等。其中质变标志明晰的文化如文字、文物、城市、礼仪等可称作文明。从唯物史观视角观察，狭义文化即精神财富，尤其体现人类精、气、神状态的事项，其本质也具有特殊物质属性，如量子也具有波粒二相性，这种粒子也是物质，无非运动方式特殊而已。现代所谓可重复验证的"科学"，事实上也是从文化中分离出来的事项，因此也是一种特殊文化形式。追求健康长寿是人类共同的夙愿。中华民族之所以繁衍昌盛，是因为健康文化异彩纷呈。中华优秀传统医药文化之所以博大精深，是因为其原创思维博大、格物致知精深，所以，习总书记说："中医药学是中国古代科学的瑰宝，也是打开中华文明宝库的钥匙"。

文化既反映时代、地域、民族分布、生产资料来源、技术水平等信息，又反映人类认知水平和生存智慧。发掘解读文物、文献中蕴藏的健康知识和灵动智慧，首先是从事健康工作者的责任和义务。《易经》设有"观"卦，人类作为观察者，不仅要积极收藏展陈文物，而且要善于捕捉文物倾诉的信息，汲取养分，启迪思维，收到古为今用之效果。墨子三表法，首先一表即"本之于古者圣王之事"，也是强调古代史实的重要性。"历史是现实的根源"，现实是未来的基础。任何一个国家、地区、民族都不能割断历史、忽略基础，这个基础就是文化。"文化是民族的血脉，是人民的精神家园"。文化繁荣才能驱动各项事业发展，才能实现中华民族的伟大复兴。

人类从类人猿分化出来。"禄丰古猿禄丰种"是云南禄丰发现的类人猿化石，距今七八百万年。距今200万年前人类进入旧石器时代，直立行走，打制石器产生工具意识，管理火种，是所谓"燧人氏"时代。中国留存有更新世早、中期的元谋、蓝田、北京人等遗址。距今10万—5万年前，人类进入旧石器时代中期，即早期智人阶段，脑容量增加，和欧洲、非洲人种相比，原始蒙古人种颧骨前突等，是所谓"伏羲氏"时代。中国发现的马坝、长阳、丁村人等较典型。距今5万—1万年前，人类进入旧石器时代晚期，即晚期智人阶段，细石器、骨角器等遍布全国，山顶洞、柳江、资阳人等较典型。

中石器时代距今约1万年，是旧石器时代向新石器时代的短暂过渡期，弓箭发明，狗被驯化。河南灵井、陕西沙苑遗址等作为代表。距今1万—公元前2600年前后，人类进入新石器时代，磨光石器、烧制陶器，出现农业村落并饲养家畜，是所谓"神农氏"时代。公元前7000年以来，在甲、骨、陶、石等载体上出现契刻符号、七音阶骨笛乐器等，反映出人文气息趋浓。公元前6000—公元前3500年的老官台、裴李岗、河姆渡、马家浜、仰韶等文化遗址，彰显出先民围绕生存健康问题所做的各种努力。

公元前4800年以来，以关中、晋南、豫西为中心形成的仰韶文化，是中原史前文化的重要标志。以半坡、庙底沟类型为典型，自公元前3500年走向繁荣，属于锄耕粟黍稻兼营渔猎饲养猪鸡经济方式，彩陶尤其发达。公元前4400—公元前3300年，长江中游的大溪文化，薄胎彩陶和白陶发达。公元前4300—公元前2500年山东丰岛的大汶口文化，红陶为主。公元前3500年前后，辽东的红山文化原始宗教发展。公元前 3300 年以来，长江下游由河姆渡、马家浜文化衍续的良渚文化和陇西的马家窑文化、江淮间的薛家岗文化时趋发达。

公元前 2600—公元前 2000 年，黄河中下游龙山文化群形成，冶铸铜器，制作玉器，土坯、石灰、夯筑技术开始应用。公元前 2697 年，轩辕战败炎帝（有说其后裔）、蚩尤而为黄帝纪元元年。黄帝西巡访贤，"至岐见岐伯，引载而归，访于治道"。其引归地"溱洧襟带于前，梅泰环拱于后"，即今河南新密市古城寨。岐黄答问，构建《黄帝内经》健康知识体系，中华文明从关注民生健康起步。颛顼改革宗教，神职人员出现；帝喾修身节用，帝尧和合百国，舜同律度量衡，大禹疏导治水，中华民族不断繁衍昌盛。

公元前 2070 年，禹之子启以豫西晋南为中心建立夏王朝，二里头青铜文化为其特征，半地穴、窑洞、地面建筑并存。饮食卫生器具、酒器增多。朱砂安神作用在宫殿应用。公元前 1600 年，商灭夏。偃师商城设有铸铜作坊。公元前 1300 年，盘庚迁殷，使用甲骨文。武丁时期青铜浑铸、分铸并存。公元前 1056 年，相传周"文王被殷纣拘于羑里，演《周易》，成六十四卦"。公元前 1046 年，武王克商建周，定都镐京。青铜器始铸长篇铭文，周原发掘出微型甲骨文字。公元前 770 年，平王东迁。虢国铸铜柄铁剑。公元前 753 年，秦国设置史官。公元前 707 年出现蝗灾、公元前 613 年出现"哈雷彗星"，均被孔子载入《春秋》。公元前 221 年，秦始皇统一中国，多元一体民族大家庭形成，中华医药卫生文物异彩纷呈。

中国是治史大国，历来重视发展文化博物事业，1955 年成立卫生部中医研究院时就设置医史研究室，1982 年中国医史文献研究所成立时复建中国医史博物馆研究收藏展陈文物。2000—2003 年，经王永炎院士、姚乃礼院长等呼吁，科技部批准立项，由李经纬、梁峻为负责人的团队完成"国家重点医药卫生文物收集调研和保护"项目任务，受到科技部项目验收组专家的高度评价，获中华中医药学会科技进步二等奖。2013 年，在国家出版基金资助下，课题组对部分文物重新拍摄或必要置换、充实民族医药文物后，由西安交通大学出版社编辑、组聘国内一流翻译团队英译说明文字付梓，受到国家中医药博物馆筹备工作领导小组和办公室的高度重视。

"物以类聚"，《图典》主要依据文物质地、种类分为 9 卷，计有陶瓷，金属，纸质，竹木，玉石、织品及标本，壁画石刻及遗址，少数民族文物，其他，备考等卷。同卷下主要根据历史年代或小类分册设章。每卷下的历史时段不求统一。遵循上述规则将《图典》划分为21册，总计收载文物5000余件。对每件文物的描述，除质地、规格、馆藏等基本要素外，重点描述其在民生健康中的作用。对少数暂不明确的事项在括号中注明待考。对引自各博物馆的材料除在文物后列出馆藏外，还在书后再次统一列出馆名或参考书目，以充分尊重其馆藏权，也同时维护本典作者的引用权。

21世纪，围绕人类健康的生命科学将飞速发展，但科学离不开文化，文化离不开文物。发掘文物承载的信息为现实服务，谨引用横渠先生四言之两语："为天地立心，为生民立命"，既作为编撰本《图典》之宗旨，也是我们践行国家"一带一路"倡议的具体努力。希冀通过本《图典》的出版发行，教育国人，提振中华民族精神；走向世界，为人类健康事业贡献力量。

李经纬　梁峻　刘学春

2017年6月于北京

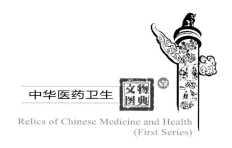

中华医药卫生 文物图典

Relics of Chinese Medicine and Health
(First Series)

目 录

1

第二章　遗址

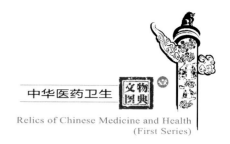

中华医药卫生 文物图典

Relics of Chinese Medicine and Health
(First Series)

Contents

Chapter Two   Historical Sites

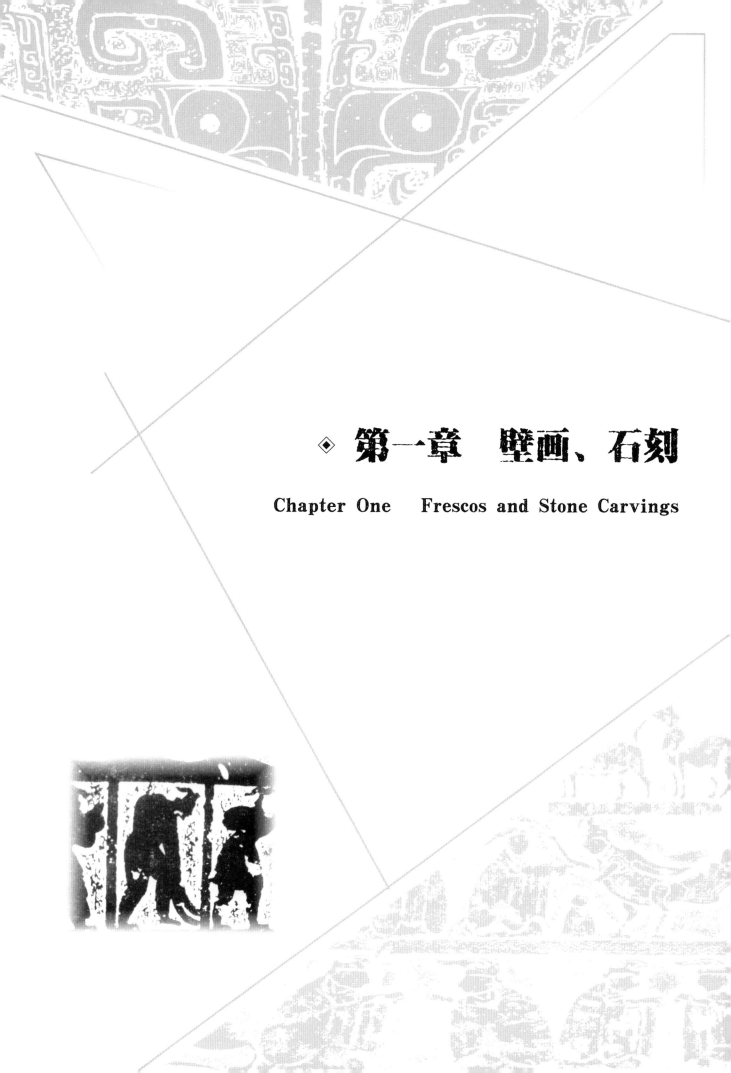

◇ 第一章　壁画、石刻

Chapter One　Frescos and Stone Carvings

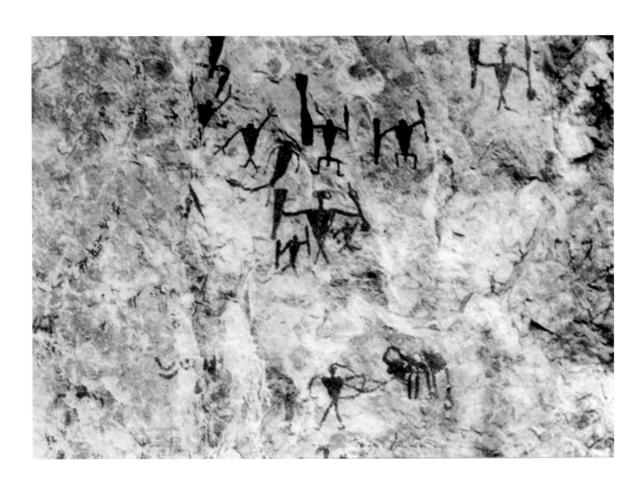

技击图岩画

青铜时代

岩画

Rock Painting of Martial Arts

Bronze Age

Rock Painting

这是一组表现人持器械进行技击演练内容的
岩画，图中人物均一手持刀，一手执盾，
呈技击状。该岩画反映了当地少数民族习
武练艺的情景。

云南省临沧市沧源县第 6 地点 6 区岩画

The painting shows a group of people practicing
martial arts with weapons. All the figures, with
a knife in one hand and a shield in the other,
are practicing attacking and defending, which
depicts the scenes of military trainings of the
local minority people.

No. 6 in Area 6, Cangyuan County, Lincang
City, Yunnan Province

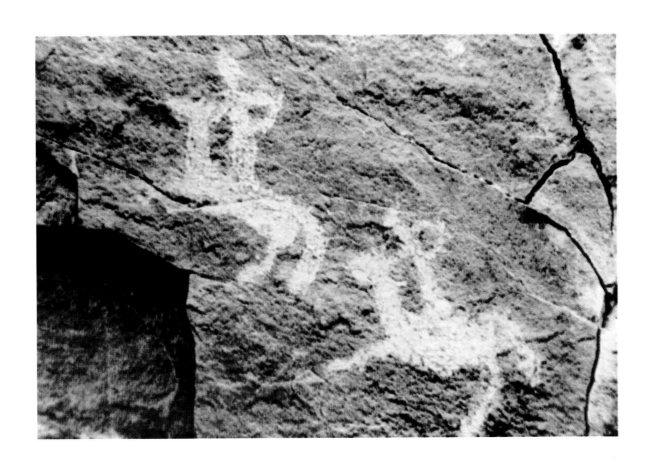

赛马图岩画

公元前 7—前 2 世纪

岩画

纵 15 厘米，横 37 厘米

Rock Painting of Horse Racing

Seven Century B.C. –Second Century B.C.

Rock Painting

Width 15 cm/ Length 37 cm

岩画凿刻在山腰上，两个骑者各骑一马，正在奋力进行赛马比赛。

内蒙古自治区巴彦淖尔市乌拉特中旗乌兰结拉嘎第 3 组岩画

Chiseled on a cliff at the mountainside, the rock painting shows two riders on horseback competing hard in a race.

No. 3 Rock Painting in Wu Lan Jie La Ga, Middle Urat Banner, Bayan Nur City, Inner Mongolia Autonomous Region

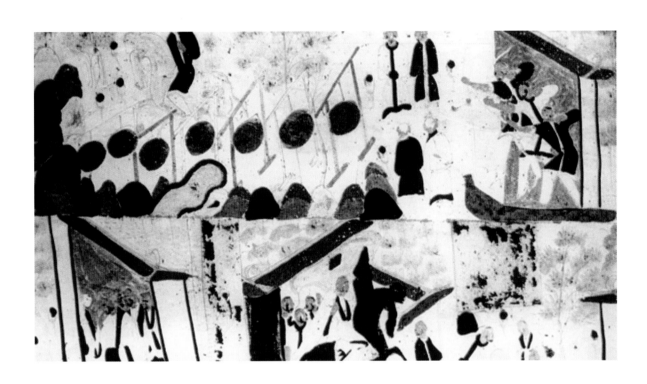

太子较射图

西周

壁画

Fresco of the Crown Prince at Shooting Competition

Western Zhou Dynasty

Fresco

壁画绘于窟内西坡的上层。内容描述的是须
达拿太子为向善觉国王的女儿求婚而应约比
试箭法的故事。图中，左侧七面铁鼓并排悬
在架上以为箭靶，右侧三位青年张弓欲射铁
鼓，旁边站立几位侍从，表现了当时射箭比
赛的真实场景。

甘肃敦煌莫高窟第 290 窟壁画

The fresco, located on the upper part of the
western slope of the grotto, tells the story of
the Crown Prince Sudana competing in arrow
shooting in order to propose to the princess
of the Kingdom of Shanjue. The fresco fully
shows the real scene of archery competition
at that time. On the left of the painting, seven
iron drums are hung side by side on a shelf
as targets; on the right, three young men are
drawing the bow to shoot with several servants
standing beside them.

In Cave 290, Mogao Grottoes, Dunhuang City,
Gansu Province

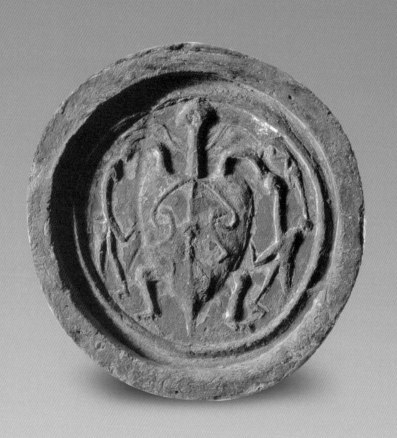

龟蛇雁纹瓦当

西汉

陶质

直径 15.7 厘米

当面中间浮雕一龟，龟两旁各有一雁，龟颈
下匍匐一条蛇。

陕西省淳化县文化馆藏

Carved Eaves Tile with Patterns of a Turtle, a Snake and Wild Geese

Western Han Dynasty

Pottery

Diameter 15.7 cm

In the tile center lies a carved turtle, which is
accompanied by a wild goose on either side and
a creeping snake under its neck.

Preserved in Chunhua Cultural Center, Shaanxi
Province

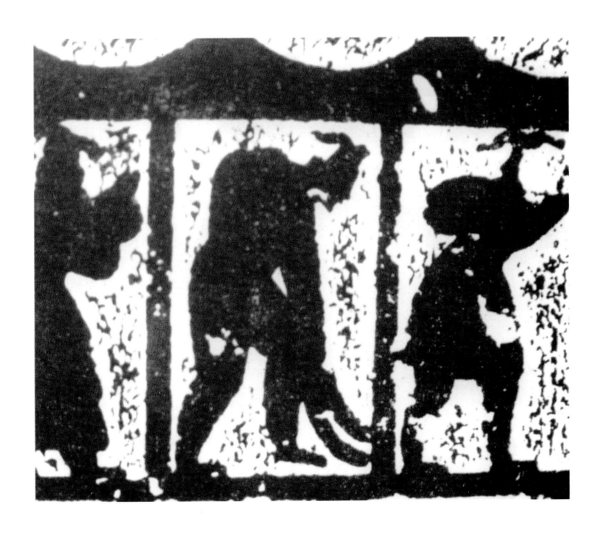

武氏祠神农氏像

东汉

画像石

Picture of Shennong in Wu's Ancestral Hall

Eastern Han Dynasty

Rock Painting

该祠建于东汉元嘉元年 (151), 现尚存画像石
5 块。此画中间一人头戴斜顶进贤冠、手持
耜呈翻地状者为神农氏。

　　山东省济宁市嘉祥县武梁祠西壁壁画

In Wu's Ancestral Hall, which was built in the
first year (151) of Yuanjia Period in Eastern
Han Dynasty, there still exist five pieces of
portrait stones. In the middle of the picture, a
man wearing a tilted Jinxian virtue man crown
is turning over the soil with a spade-shaped
farm tool Si. He is recognized as Shennong, the
inventor of Chinese farming and medicine.
On the western wall of Wu's Ancestral Hall
in Jiaxiang County, Jining City, Shandong
Province

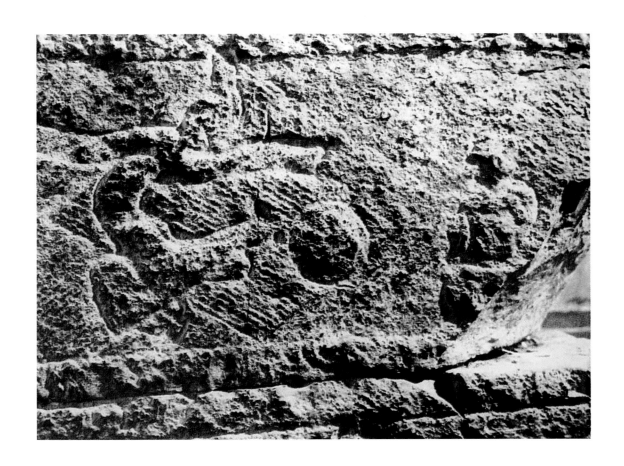

蹴鞠图画像石局部

东汉

画像石

原石：纵 37 厘米，横 100 厘米

Relief Stone with Cuju Ball Kicking Design

Eastern Han Dynasty

Stone Carving

Original Stone: Width 37 cm/ Length 100 cm

画像石位于启母阙西阙北面第五层右边，表现的是一女子蹴鞠的形象。画像中蹴鞠女动态优美，活泼可爱，具有舞蹈的韵律感。从其旁边的伴奏者来看，这一画面反映的应是一表演性质的蹴鞠活动。

河南省登封市嵩山启母阙画像石

The relief stone is on the right part of the fifth level on the northern wall of the western Qimu Tower. It displays a woman kicking cuju ball, who is elegant and vigorous, and moves with dancing rhythms. The presence of an accompanist nearby suggests that this was an entertainment performance of a cuju ball kicking.

Preserved in the Qimu Stone Carvings, Mount Song, Dengfeng City, Henan Province

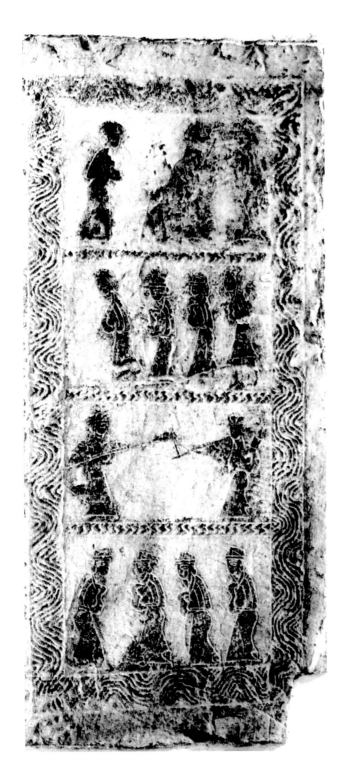

比武画像石

东汉

画像石

纵 123 厘米，横 59 厘米

Relief Stone with Carvings of Martial Arts Competition

Eastern Han Dynasty

Stone Carving

Width 123 cm/ Length 59 cm

画面共分为四格，均是围绕着比武这个主题
所展示的连续内容。其中第三格即为比武图，
左边一人执钩戟，右边一人执戈，正互相对
击。而第一、第二和第四格分别为二人相邀
观武、四人同行和三人施礼作别。江苏省徐
州市铜山区韩楼出土。

　　江苏省徐州市狮子山楚王陵内博物馆藏

The four scenes on the stone continuously
narrate the course of a martial arts competition.
The third scene demonstrates the competition
in which the man on the left with a halberd
is fighting with the right one with a lance,
while the first scene describes two men invited
to watch the competition; the second scene
illustrates four people coming to watch the
competition; and the fourth scene shows three
men giving a farewell bowing. It was unearthed
in Hanlou, Tongshan District of Xuzhou City,
Jiangsu Province.
Preserved in the museum of the Tomb of King
of Chu at Mount Shizishan, Xuzhou City

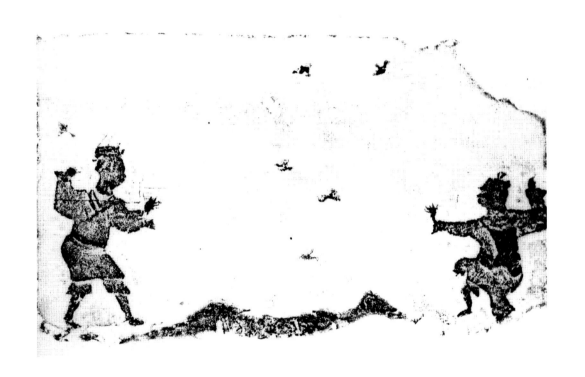

拳术画像砖拓片

东汉

画砖像

纵 27 厘米，横 45 厘米，厚 6.5 厘米

Rubbing of Relief Brick with Boxing Carving

Eastern Han Dynasty

Brick

Width 27 cm/ Length 45 cm/ Thickness 6.5 cm

画像上两人伸臂屈腕，一人半蹲，一人弯腰前倾，在田野上相对练拳。该画像砖为今存较早的有关拳术的实物资料。原砖于四川省成都市新都区出土。

四川省成都市新都区文物管理所藏

The two figures in relief are practicing boxing face to face in an open field, one squatting while the other bending forward. The brick, the earliest material object of boxing so far, was unearthed in Xindu District, Sichuan Province. Preserved in Xindu District Administration Office of Cultural Relics, Chengdu City Sichuan Province

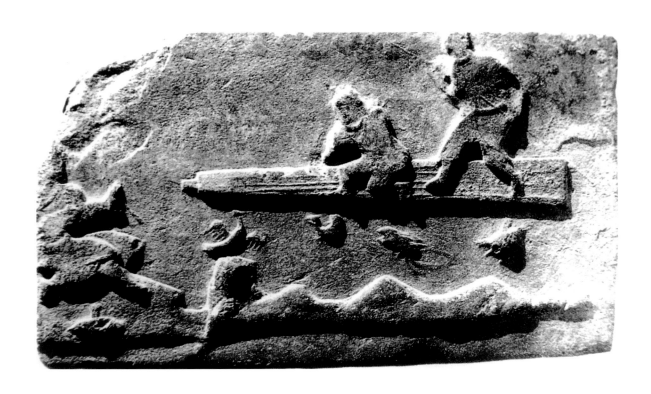

垂钓行筏画像砖

东汉

画像砖

纵 26 厘米，横 44 厘米

Relief Brick with Carving of Fishing and Rafting

Eastern Han Dynasty

Brick

Width 26 cm/ Length 44 cm

作者运用高浮雕的艺术手法，雕刻出了一幅大江行筏、渔者岸边垂钓的画面：江中的竹筏上坐着二人，一人手执长竿正在撑筏；左边的垂钓者正从水面钓出一条活蹦乱跳的鱼。寥寥数笔，勾绘出一幅意趣清新、生机盎然的人物山水画。

四川省成都市新都区文物管理所藏

The brick is carved in high relief with a drawing of rafting in the river and fishing from the river bank. Of the two men on the raft, one is propelling it with a pole. The fisherman on the left is fishing a kicking fish out of the water. Carved just with simple lines, the drawing of a landscape and figures achieves fresh taste and natural vitality.

Preserved in Xindu District Administration Office of Cultural Relics, Chengdu City, Sichuan Province

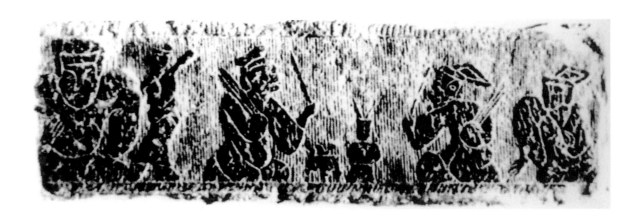

投壶画像石

东汉

画像石

纵 42 厘米，横 131 厘米

Relief Stone with Carving of Pitch-pot Game

Eastern Han Dynasty

Stone Carving

Width 42 cm/ Length 131 cm

画面中部两人，一戴平帻，一戴进贤冠，均着长衣相对踞坐，一手抱矢，一手执矢投壶，中间壶内有两矢。壶旁置一酒樽，左边两人，似正在酒后离席，右边一人在踞坐旁观。图中内容生动地再现了汉代投壶活动的盛况。

南阳汉画馆藏

In the middle part of the drawing, two men, one in a plain flat headdress and the other in a virtuous–man recommeder's crown with tassels, are sitting face to face in long dresses, pitching an arrow with one hand while holding some with the other hand. Between them stands a pot with two arrows in it and a wine bottle beside it. Two figures on the left are seemingly leaving from the banquet, while the one on the right is watching the game kneeling on the ground with his back upright. This drawing vividly displays pitch-pot games in Han Dynasty.
Preserved in Nanyang Museum of Han Dynasty Stone Reliefs

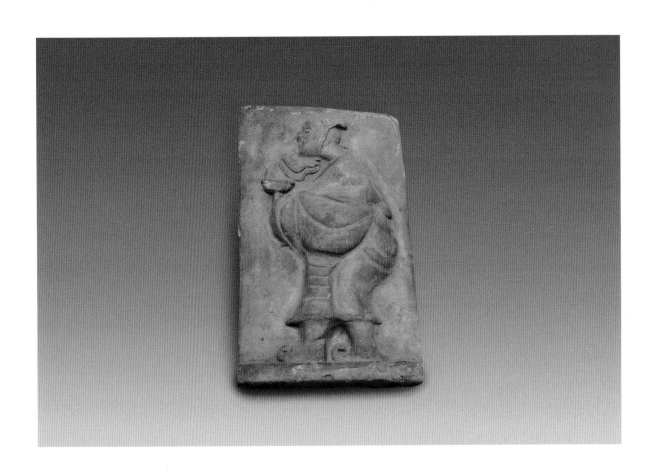

画像砖

汉

陶质

27 厘米 ×17 厘米 ×2 厘米

Relief Brick

Han Dynasty

Pottery

27 cm × 17 cm × 2 cm

画像砖为高浮雕的侍食俑图案。由学校老师
捐赠。

　　成都中医药大学中医药传统文化博物馆藏

The figure in high relief on the brick is an
attendant serving dinner. It was donated by a
teacher.

Preserved in Museum of Traditional Chinese
Medicine Culture, Chengdu University of
Traditional Chinese Medicine

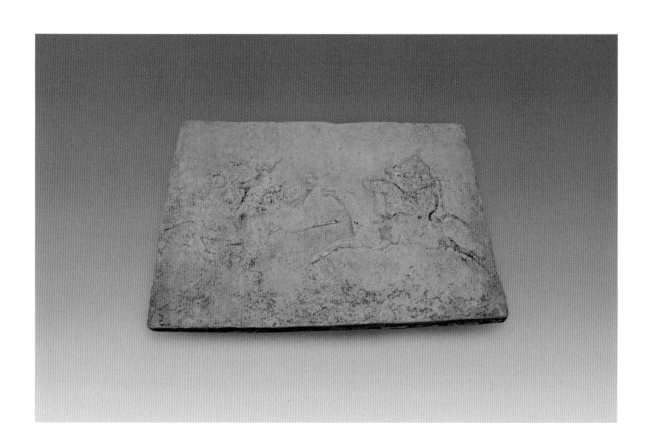

画像砖

汉

陶质

45 厘米 ×32 厘米 ×2 厘米

Relief Brick

Han Dynasty

Pottery

45 cm × 32 cm × 2 cm

画像砖为骑马射箭的图案。由学校老师捐赠。

成都中医药大学中医药传统文化博物馆藏

The brick is carved with patterns of arrow shooting on horseback. It was denoted by a teacher.

Preserved in Museum of Traditional Chinese Medicine Culture, Chengdu University of Traditional Chinese Medicine

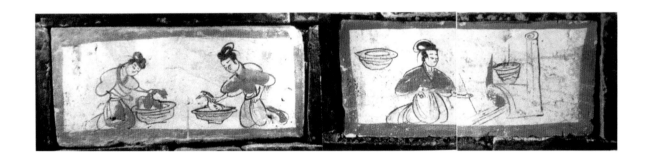

墓砖画像

魏晋

画壁砖

纵 21 厘米，横 36 厘米

Grave-brick Paintings

Wei or Jin Dynasty

Brick

Width 21 cm/ Length 36 cm

墓砖共 600 多块。砖画色彩淡雅，线条清晰，内容以描写当时的现实生活为主。图示左为烫洗家禽，右为做饭。甘肃省嘉峪关东北 20 公里的戈壁滩上出土。

甘肃省酒泉市博物馆藏

There are more than 600 bricks in total. The paintings on the bricks are lightly colored and clearly lined, mainly describing the real life at that time. The photo on the left shows the scene of cleaning poultry with hot water and the right one is about cooking. They were unearthed from the Gobi Desert, 20 km northeast away from Jiayuguan Pass, Gansu Province.

Preserved in Jiuquan Museum, Gansu Province

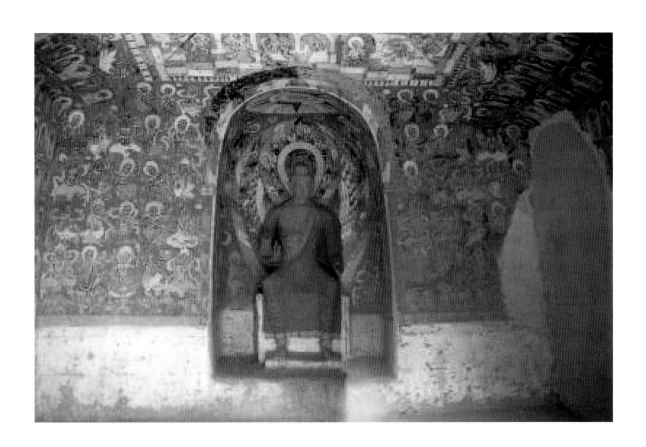

动功图

北凉

壁画

Fresco of Dynamic Exercise

Northern Liang Dynasty

Fresco

壁画共有各种动功形态的人物图像 40 幅，
分绘在洞窟正面的两侧。每侧有 20 幅画面，
各分为上下四层，每层中的每一个人动作都
不一样，连续起来，为一完整的动功图。

　　　　甘肃敦煌莫高窟第 272 窟北壁壁画

Forty paintings of figures in various dynamic
actions scatter on the wall on the two sides of
the cave. Twenty on either side, the paintings
are placed on four levels. Each individual's
movements are different from the others.
Viewed as a whole, the paintings are a complete
demonstration of some dynamic exercises.
On the northern wall in Cave No. 272, Mogao
Grottoes, Dunhuang City, Gansu Province

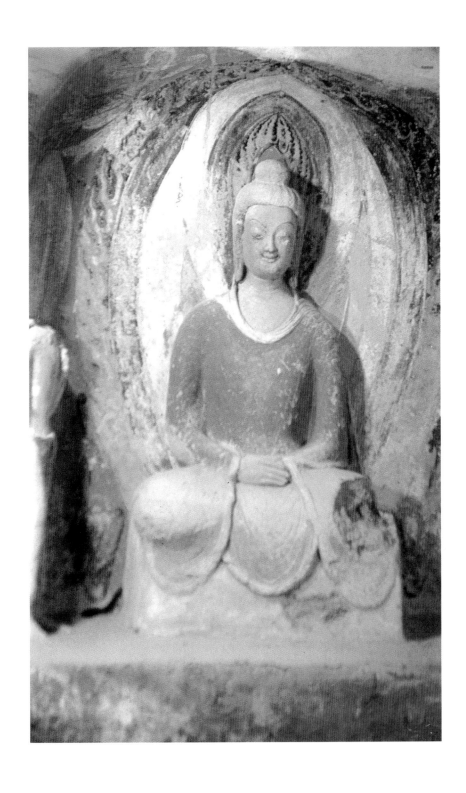

静功（坐禅）图

北魏

彩塑

佛家坐禅悟性即可视为是作静功。要求：坐禅者盘腿而坐，双手虚合，双目轻闭，心静无波，无欲无求。以吐纳、意守、内视为方法，培养真气通周天，以壮其内。

甘肃敦煌莫高窟第 259 窟北壁下层彩塑

Statue of (Zen) Meditation

Northern Wei Dynasty

Painted Clay Statue

Buddhists regard meditation as static exercise in which the practicer sits cross-legged, cups his/her palms together devoutly, closes his/her eyes slightly, and calms the mind to wipe off any desire. While meditating, one can build up the body by circulating qi (breath) within the body with the methods of inhalation and exhalation, mental concentration, and inward observation.

On the lower level of northern wall in Cave No. 259, Mogao Grottoes, Dunhuang City, Gansu Province

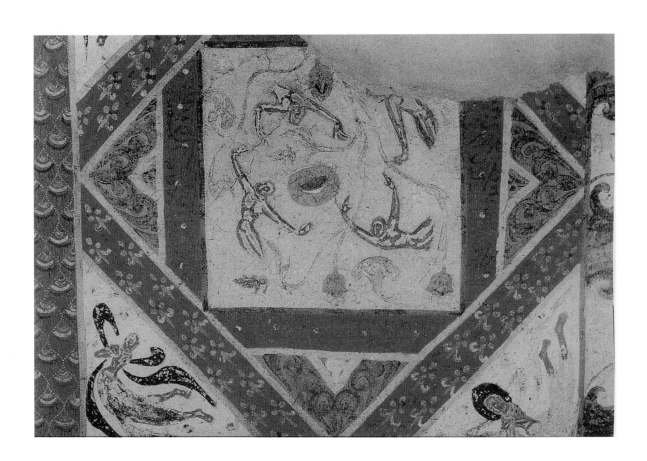

游泳图壁画

北魏

壁画

Fresco of Swimming

Northern Wei Dynasty

Fresco

游泳图绘于窟内顶部平棋图案的中心。在一碧绿的池水中，四位击水者出没起伏于莲花之间，他们的击水、浮水动作舒展有力，展示了一群喜泳者的优美姿态。

甘肃敦煌莫高窟第 257 窟壁画

Drawn on the ceiling of a grotto and framed by a square, the painting shows that four figures are swimming with vigorous motions and graceful gestures in a pool dotted with lotuses. This is truly a beautiful picture of swimming fans.
In Cave No. 257, Mogao Grottoes, Dunhuang City, Gansu Province

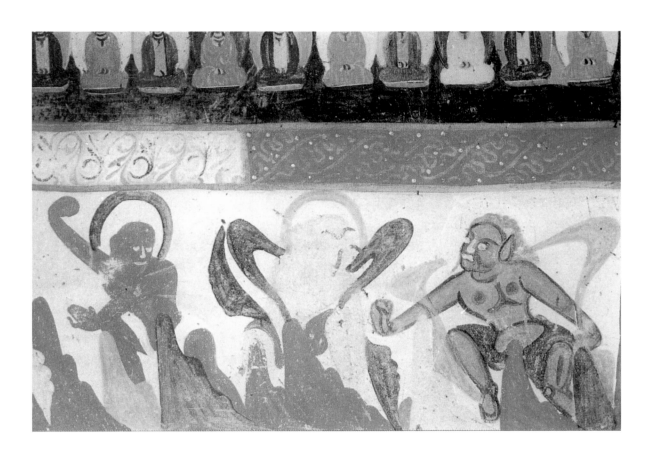

力士相搏图壁画

北魏

壁画

Fresco of Wrestling

Northern Wei Dynasty

Fresco

图中，二力士造型身体强壮，裸身仅着犊鼻裤，正在舞臂踢腿、徒手相搏，由其相搏的动作看，已显具拳术技击中的功架、程式特征。壁画绘于该窟西壁下部。

甘肃敦煌莫高窟第 251 窟壁画

Two robust men, only in crotch cloth, are extending arms and legs to wrestle, which is quite similar to martial arts in posture and procedure. The fresco is at the lower section of the western wall in the cave.

In Cave No. 251, Mogao Grottoes, Dunhuang City, Gansu Province

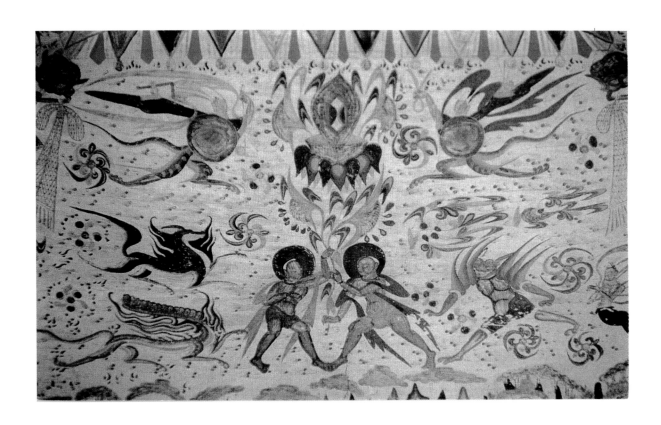

伏羲与女娲

西魏

壁画

Fresco of Fuxi and Nuwa

Western Wei Dynasty

Fresco

壁画上部为伏羲（左）和女娲（右），中国
神话中传为人类创始之神，亦为日月之神。
下部正中裸体的二力士手捧摩尼宝珠。壁画
表现了天宫诸仙与人间僧侣修道的情景。一
动一静，营造深幽的意境。

甘肃敦煌莫高窟 285 窟壁画

The figures in the upper part of the fresco are
Fuxi (on the left) and Nuwa (on the right)
who are believed to be the initial ancestors of
human beings and Sun God and Moon Goddess
in Chinese folktales. Below them stand two
strong naked men holding treasure beads in
their hands. Portraying flying gods in Heavenly
Palace and meditating monks in human's world,
the fresco creates an artistic mood with the
contrasting dynamic and static figures.
In Cave No. 285, Mogao Grottoes, Dunhuang
City, Gansu Province

相扑图浮雕

西魏

浮雕

Relief Painting of Sumo

Western Wei Dynasty

Relief Painting

该浮雕为表现佛教故事的一个画面的局部，
位于整个石刻画面的右上方。浮雕描述了两
位头戴冠、着短裤的力士正在相扑的情形。

陕西省宜君县福地水库石窟浮雕

The painting is part of a picture about a
Buddhist tale. At the right top of the relief
stone, the painting portrays two strong sumo
wrestlers with hats and short pants.
In Fudi Reservoir Grottoes, Yijun County,
Shaanxi Province

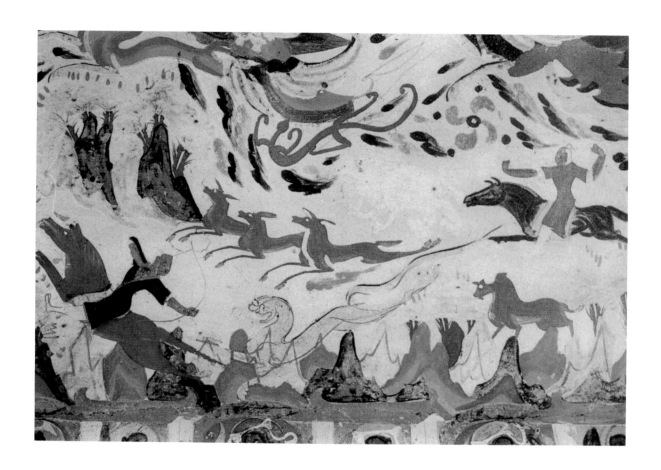

射猎图壁画

西魏

壁画

Fresco of Hunting

Western Wei Dynasty

Fresco

图中山峦叠嶂，树木丛生，右上角一骑士身骑奔马，双臂呈拉弓状对准前方的猎物；左下角的骑士正返身执弓射向迎面扑来的猛虎。画面中射手、动物、背景融为一体，具有较强的运动感。此图绘于窟内主室北披。

甘肃敦煌莫高窟第 249 窟壁画

Among the rolling woody mountains, the rider on a galloping horse on the upper right of the fresco is drawing the bow at his prey ahead. The rider on the lower left is turning round and shooting at a fierce tiger jumping at him. Integrating the hunter and prey into the background, the painting exhibits a strong dynamic sense. It is on the northern wall of the main chamber in the cave.

In Cave No. 249, Mogao Grottoes, Dunhuang City, Gansu Province

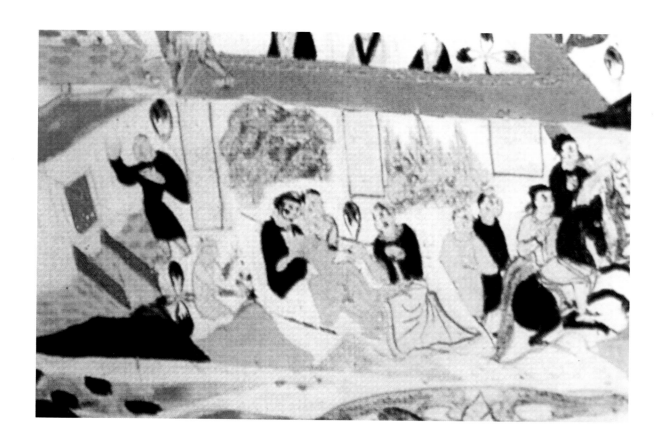

诊病施药图

北周

壁画

Fresco of Diagnosis and Medication

Northern Zhou Dynasty

Fresco

这是《福田经变》画的一个场面：两位家属扶着半躺的瘦弱的患者，医生在右侧正在为患者认真地检查诊断，左侧一人在用药臼捣制药物。

甘肃敦煌莫高窟 296 窟壁画

The fresco describes a scene recorded in "Fu Tian Jing Bian" (*Illustration of Happiness Field Sutra*): a doctor on the right is attentively diagnosing a weak patient who is reclining and supported by two of his family members, and the man on the left is grinding medicine with a mortar and pestle.

In Cave No. 296, Mogao Grottoes, Dunhuang City, Gansu Province

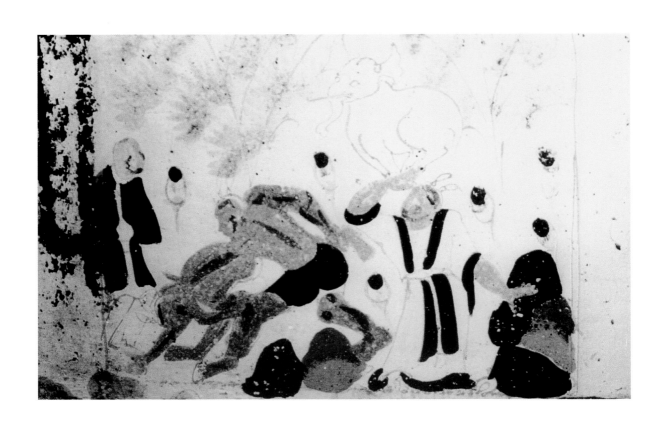

相扑图壁画

北周

壁画

Fresco of Sumo

Northern Zhou Dynasty

Fresco

《相扑图》在窟内西披上层，为佛传故事画内容之一。图中，须达拿太子左手拿住大力魔王脖颈，右手抓住其右脚踩，正要将其抛翻在地。相扑双方均赤裸上身，下着短裤，体态强壮，人物造型显得拙朴生动。

甘肃敦煌莫高窟第 290 窟壁画

At the upper part of the western wall, the fresco tells a Buddhist tale. Crown Prince Sudana is throwing the Strong Devil down to the ground, choking him by the neck with his left hand, and grabbing his right ankle with his right hand. These two massively built wrestlers, bare to the waist but in shorts, are portrayed plainly but vividly.

In Cave No. 290, Mogao Grottoes, Dunhuang City, Gansu Province

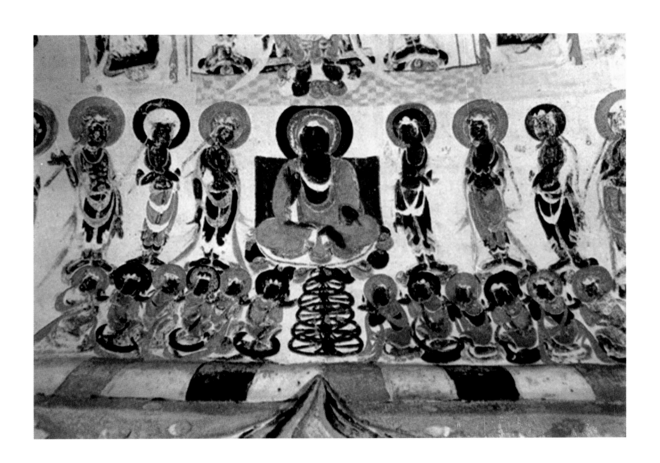

药师经变

隋

壁画

Fresco of the Illustration of the Medicine Buddha Sutra

Sui Dynasty

Fresco

居中莲台上结跏趺坐为药师琉璃光佛，又称
大医王佛，居东方净琉璃世界，发十二大愿，
救众生之病源，治无名之痼疾。两侧各侍立
菩萨四身，为药师八大菩萨。

甘肃敦煌莫高窟第 417 窟壁画

Medicine Guru Buddha, also called Medicine
Buddha Bhaishajyaguru, is sitting in lotus
position on the middle lotus seat. He lives in the
Pure Land of the East and issues twelve vows
in order to save all living creatures' lives and
cure unknown chronic diseases. There are four
Bodhisattvas standing respectively on his two
sides who are known as the eight Bodhisattvas
of Medicine Buddha.

In Cave No. 417, Mogao Grottoes, Dunhuang
City, Gansu Province

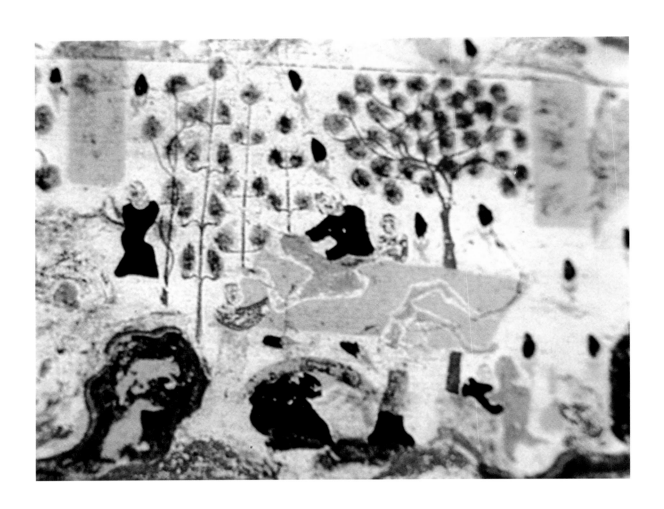

正骨图

隋

壁画

Fresco of Bone-setting

Sui Dynasty

Fresco

壁画为窟顶人字坡西坡下端《福田经变》中
的治疗场面。患者裸体卧席上，家属二人各
执其左右手，医生正对患者进行正骨治疗。

甘肃敦煌莫高窟第 302 窟壁画

This fresco is about the treatment scene in "Fu Tian Jing Bian" (*Illustration of Happiness Field Sutra*) at the lower end of the western herringbone slope of the grotto top. The naked patient is lying on the mat. His two family members are grasping his two hands, and the doctor is setting his bone.

In Cave No. 302, Mogao Grottoes, Dunhuang City, Gansu Province

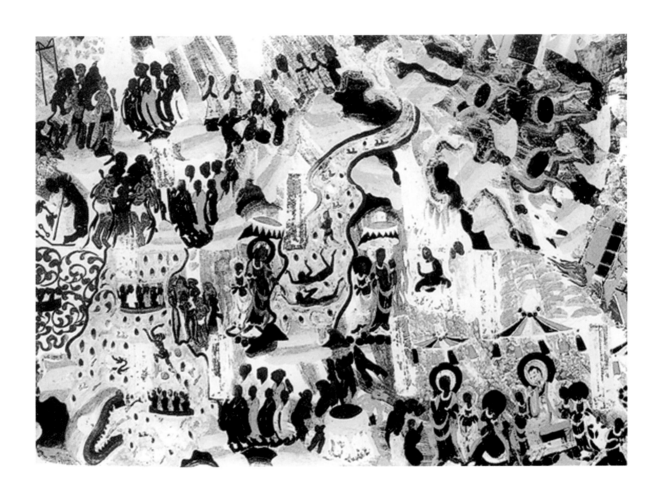

游泳图壁画

隋

壁画

Fresco of Swimming

Sui Dynasty

Fresco

游泳图绘于窟内覆斗形藻井东坡。其表现的是佛教中观世音拯救诸般苦难，包括溺水者的情景。画面中部的河水中，溺水者并不呈惊慌失措之态，反被刻画成了活泼健美、生气勃勃的善泳者的形象。

甘肃敦煌莫高窟第 420 窟壁画

This fresco is on the eastern slope of the upturned bucket-shaped caisson. It expresses the scene of Avalokitesvara's rescuing various sufferings, including rescuing a drowning man. But the drowning man in the river in the middle of the painting does not look panic-stricken. On the contrary, he is depicted as a good swimmer who is active, strong and spirited.

In Cave No. 420, Mogao Grottoes, Dunhuang City, Gansu Province

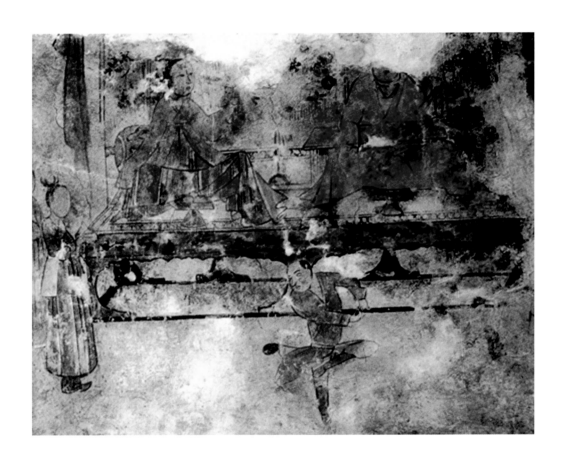

宴享伎乐图壁画

隋

壁画

纵 75 厘米，横 94 厘米

Fresco of Enjoying Music and Show at the Banquet

Sui Dynasty

Fresco

Width 75 cm/ Length 94 cm

此图绘于隋开皇四年 (584) 徐敏行墓墓室北壁。图中徐氏夫妇举杯相敬，榻前有鼓吹乐人，庭中踢球人身着胡服，球用绳系于腰间，两目注视踢起之球，一腿曲盘上踢，两手起舞，似与鼓乐和拍按节而动。其全神贯注之状，使观者神往。1976年山东省嘉祥县杨楼村出土。

山东省吉祥县徐敏行墓壁画

This fresco is on the northern wall of the coffin chamber, painted in the Fourth Year of Kaihuang Period of the Sui Dynasty (584) .In the painting, Xu Minxing and his wife are proposing a toast to each other. There are minstrels playing wind and drum music in front of their couch. In the middle of the hall, a player who wears Hufu clothing is kicking the ball that is tied around his waist by a rope. He looks at the rising ball with one of his legs bending upward. He raises his hands, seemingly dancing to the drum. He is so absorbed in playing that the onlookers are all charmed with it. It was unearthed in 1976 in Yanglou Village, Jiaxiang County, Shandong Province.

In Xu Minxing's Grave, Jiaxiang County, Shandong Province

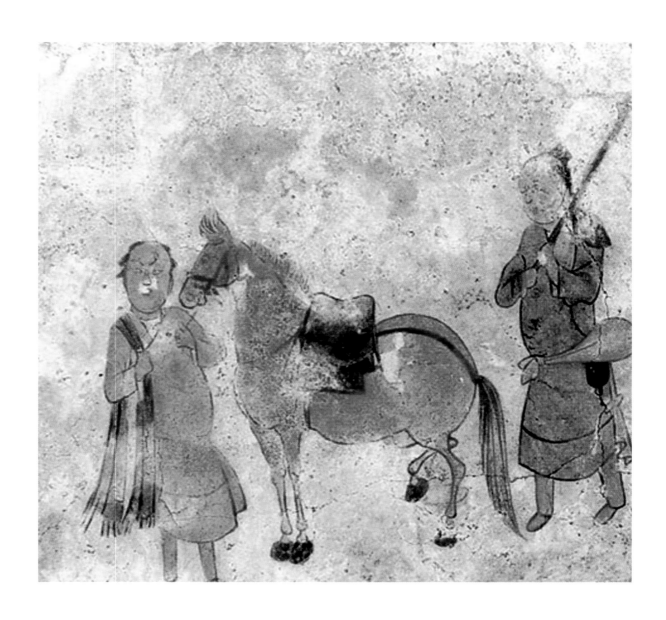

备骑图壁画

隋

壁画

纵 70 厘米，横 107 厘米

壁画绘于隋开皇四年（584）徐敏行墓墓室西壁。图中二人一马伫立待行。马已备鞍，马前一人执马缰在顾盼，马后一人双手持鞠杖相随，再现了马球比赛前的生动场景。1976 年山东省嘉祥县杨楼村出土。

山东省嘉祥县除敏行墓壁画

Fresco of Preparing for Polo Riding

Sui Dynasty

Fresco

Width 70 cm/ Length 107 cm

The fresco is on the western wall of the coffin chamber, painted in the Fourh Year of Kaihuang Period of the Sui Dynasty (584). In the painting, two men and a horse are standing and are ready for setoff. The horse has already been saddled. The man in front of the horse is looking around with the bridle rein in his hand, and the other man standing behind the horse is following with a ball rod in his hands. The painting reproduces the lively scene of preparation for a polo game at that time. It was unearthed in 1976 in Yanglou Village, Jiaxiang County, Shandong Province.

In Xu Minxing's Grave, Jiaxiang County, Shandong Province

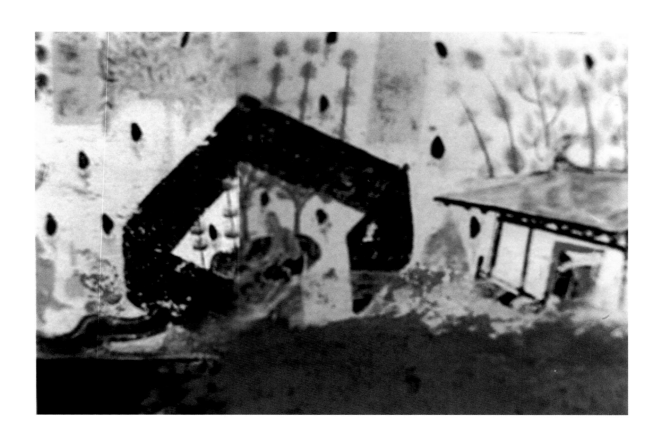

洗浴图

隋

壁画

Fresco of Bathing

Sui Dynasty

Fresco

两个裸体的人在四周有树木的浴池内洗澡。《佛传故事》中的九龙口吐泉水，为太子沐浴，宛如一幅慈母在龙头装饰的淋浴下为儿童洗浴的写实画。其采自敦煌莫高窟302窟的《福田经变》。

甘肃敦煌莫高窟第302窟壁画

In the painting, two naked men are bathing in a bathing pool which is surrounded by trees. The painting vividly describes a story in *Buddhist Tales* of a crown prince's bathing under the spring water running from the nine dragons' mouths. It is just like a mother bathing her child under a dragon head-shaped shower head. It is one of the frescoes of "Fu Tian Jing Bian" (*Illustration of Happiness Field Sutra*) in Cave No. 302, Mogao Grottoes, Dunhuang.

In Cave No. 302, Mogao Grottoes, Dunhuang City, Gansu Province

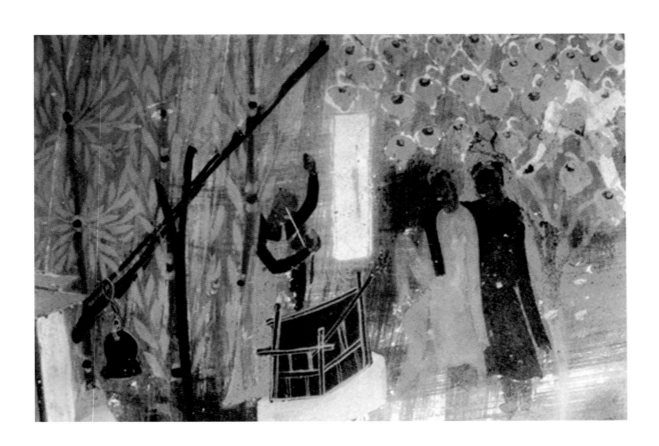

拦护水井图

隋

壁画

Fresco of Fenced Well

Sui Dynasty

Fresco

敦煌莫高窟 419 窟中须达拿本生故事画及
296 窟、302 窟的两幅《福田经变》，所绘
水井上都有围栏，有保护饮水清洁及增强安
全性的作用。

甘肃敦煌莫高窟第 419 窟壁画

Wells in the paintings of Crown Prince Sudana's
stories in Grotto No. 419 and the other two
paintings of "Fu Tian Jing Bian" (*Illustration
of Happiness Field Sutra*) in Grotto No. 296
and Grotto No. 302 are all fenced. Fences could
keep the drinking water clean and make it safer.
In Cave No. 419, Mogao Grottoes, Dunhuang
City, Gansu Province

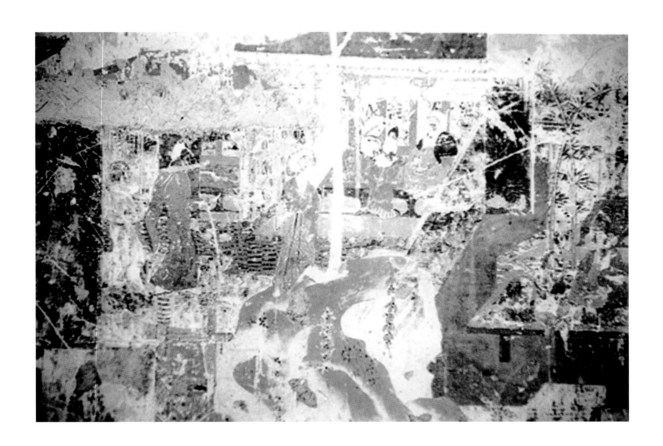

得医图

唐

壁画

Fresco of Medical Treatment

Tang Dynasty

Fresco

壁画系根据《妙法莲七经·第 22 卷》中的"如病得医"四字描绘的医疗场景。其采自敦煌莫高窟第 217 窟。

甘肃中医药大学中国医学史博物馆藏

This fresco is about the scene of medical treatment described by the four Chinese characters "Ru Bing De Yi" in *The Wonderful Dharma Lotus Flower Sutra* (Vol. 22), which mean "as one can get medical treatment when he is ill". It is from the Cave No. 217, Mogao Grottoes, Dunhuang.

Preserved in the Museum of Chinese Medicine History, Gansu University of Chinese Medicine

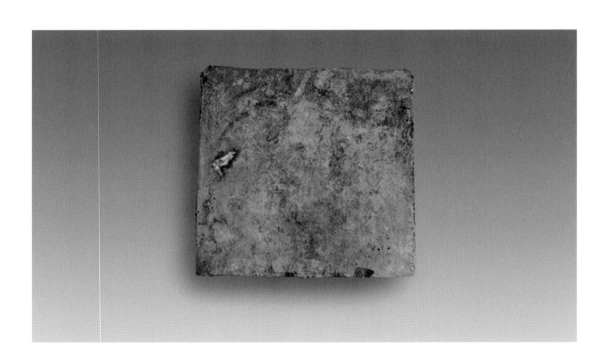

崔庭珪墓志铭

唐

石质

33 厘米 ×33 厘米 ×9 厘米

Cui Tinggui's Epitaph

Tang Dynasty

Stone

33 cm × 33 cm × 9 cm

该墓志铭为正方形。文字内容简要地介绍了崔庭珪的身世。该石为陪葬品，三级文物，完整无损。1986 年入藏，陕西省西安市长安区征集。

陕西医史博物馆藏

This square-shaped gravestone is a burial object. The words on it are the brief introduction of Cui Tinggui's life experience. It was collected in 1986 in Chang'an District Xi'an City, Shaanxi Province. It is a third-class cultural relic and is still in good condition.

Preserved in Shaanxi Museum of Medical History

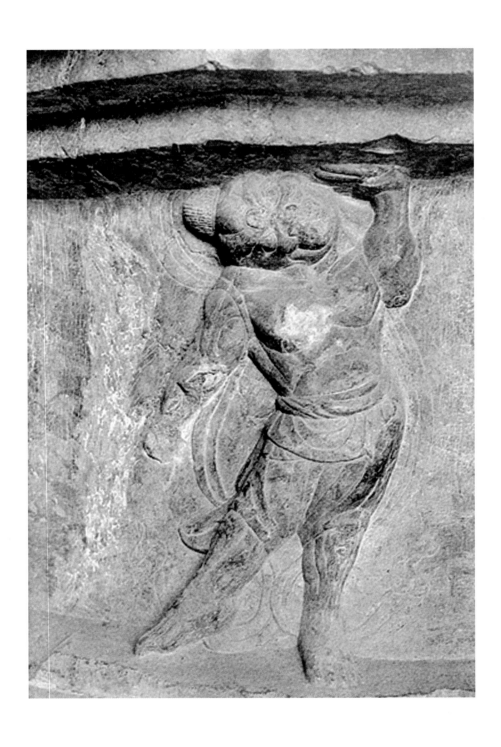

托举力士石雕

唐

石雕

高 47 厘米

力士仰首托掌奋力承托。其上体袒裸，胸、腹肌肉刻画入微。上身之帔帛飘荡，下身之战裙飞扬，瞪目闭唇，其形态极为生动。

河南洛阳龙门石窟万佛洞西壁雕像

Stone Carving of the Weightlifting Man

Tang Dynasty

Stone Carving

Height 47 cm

The weightlifting man is raising his head and does all he could to support the upper part. His upper body is naked. The muscles on his chest and stomach are portrayed to life. The short embroidered cape he wears is fluttering, and the war skirt is flying. He closes his mouth and opens his eyes, which is supremely lively.

On the western wall of Ten-thousand Buddhas Cave in Longmen Grottoes, Luoyang City, Henan Province

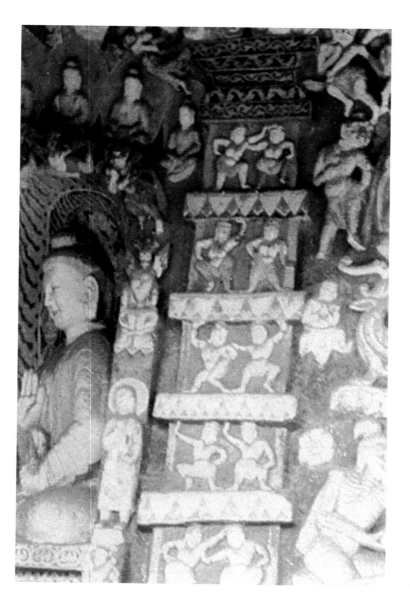

双人对练图浮雕

唐

浮雕

Embossment of Paired Exercise

Tang Dynasty

Embossment

这是第 7 窟内的一幅浮雕。在一立柱上分五层雕有五组双人赤手对练图。画面形象反映了当时人们对练习武的真实情景。

山西大同云冈石窟浮雕

This embossment is in the seventh grotto. Five pairs of people are carved on five tiers on a vertical column. The painting vividly reflects the real scene of exercising martial arts in pairs at that time.

Yungang Grottoes, Datong City, Shanxi Province

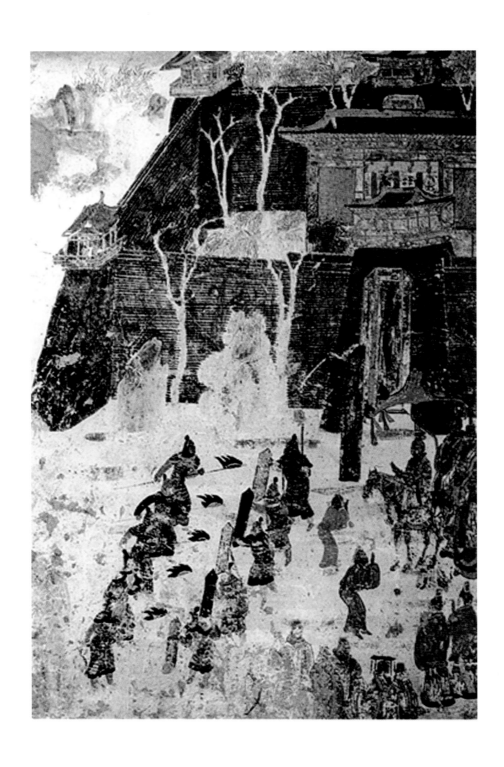

对练图壁画

唐

壁画

画面背景为一城堡，城堡外的空地上，十位武士分两列，一列武士执枪对刺，一列武士执刀、盾相迎。图中所展示的是一武术器械对练的场景。

甘肃敦煌莫高窟第 217 窟壁画

Fresco of Paired Exercise

Tang Dynasty

Fresco

The background of the picture is a castle, in front of which ten warriors in two rows are doing paired exercises. One row of them is bayoneting with spears, while the other row of warriors is meeting them with swords and shields. The painting shows the scene of paired exercise of armed martial arts.

In Cave No. 217, Mogao Grottoes, Dunhuang City, Gansu Province

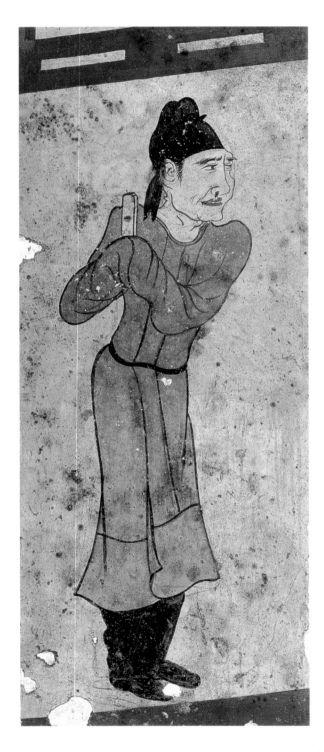

持笏给使图

唐

壁画

人物高 104 厘米

Painting of a Gei Shi Holding a Hu

Tang Dynasty

Fresco

Height of the Figure 104 cm

给使，即被阉割了的男侍。在封建社会里，这类人物除了宫廷宦官外，还出现在一些朝廷重臣和外命妇的府邸。作者用夸张的手法反映给使因阉割而造成的形体变化和奴颜婢膝的心理状态。

陕西昭陵博物馆藏

Gei Shi is a castrated man for service in ancient China. In the feudal society, these people served not only in the palace but also in the mansions of high-ranking officials and court-honored prestigious women living far away from the capital. The painter depicts the deformity and servility of the castrated man in an exaggerated manner.

Preserved in Zhao Tomb Museum of Shaanxi Province

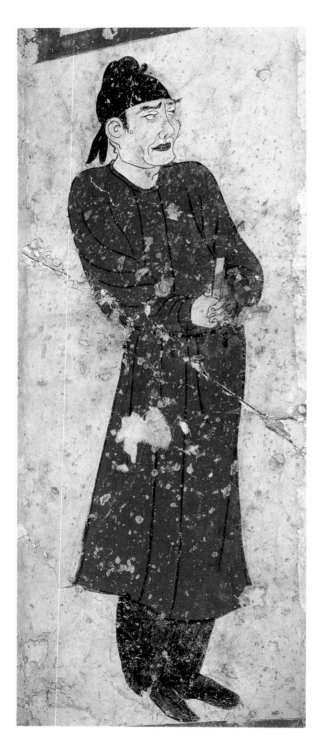

持笏给使图

唐

壁画

人物高 106 厘米

Painting of a Gei Shi Holding a Hu

Tang Dynasty

Fresco

Height of the Figure 106 cm

给使，即被阉割了的男侍。在封建社会里，这类人物除了宫廷宦官外，还出现在一些朝廷重臣和外命妇的府邸。作者用夸张的手法反映给使因阉割而造成的形体变化和奴颜婢膝的心理状态。

陕西昭陵博物馆藏

Gei Shi is a castrated man for service in ancient China. In the feudal society, these people served not only in the palace but also in the mansions of high-ranking officials and court-honored prestigious women living away from the capital. The painter depicts the deformity and servility of the castrated man in an exaggerated manner.
Preserved in Zhao Tomb Museum of Shaanxi Province

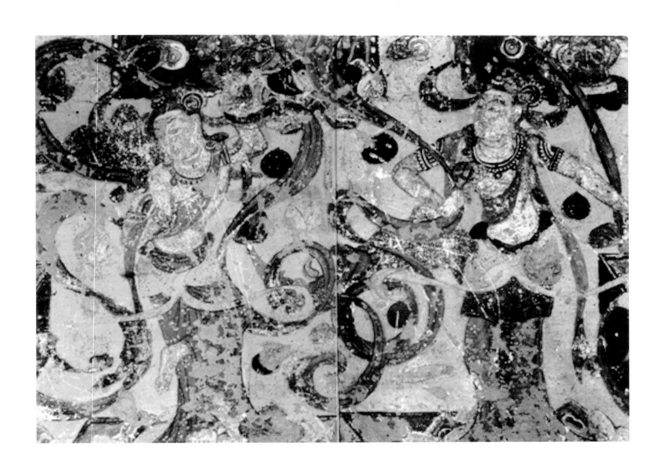

舞蹈图

唐
壁画

Fresco of Dancing

Tang Dynasty

Fresco

此图为壁画中少见的拓枝舞，舞者手执长带，
在莲花上急速旋转。

甘肃敦煌莫高窟第 217 窟北壁壁画

It is quite rare to see Tuozhi dance in frescoes.
In this painting of a Tuozhi dance, dancers with
strips in their hands are spinning quickly on
lotus flowers.
On the northern wall of Cave No. 217, Mogao
Grottoes, Dunhuang City, Gansu Province

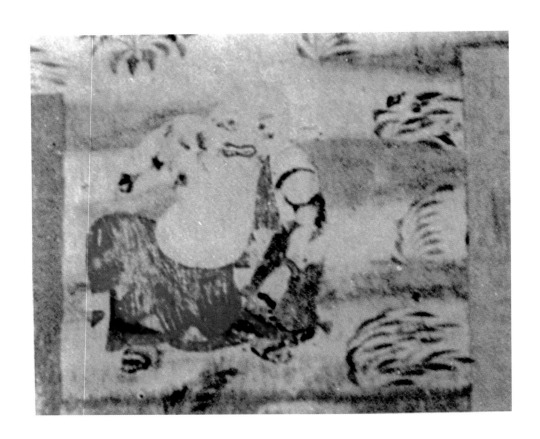

揩牙图

唐
壁画

Fresco of Wiping Teeth

Tang Dynasty

Fresco

一个受戒者剃光了头蹲在地上，左手拿着漱口的水瓶，右手中指揩其前齿。采自敦煌莫高窟 196 窟之《劳度叉斗圣变》图。

甘肃敦煌莫高窟第 196 窟壁画

In the painting, an ordained monk is squatting on the ground, holding a water bottle in his left hand. He is wiping his incisors with the middle finger of his right hand. It is one of the frescoes of "Lao Du Cha Dou Sheng Bian" (*Illustration of Raudraksa's Battle Sutra*) in Cave No. 196, Mogao Grottoes, Dunhuang.

In Cave No. 196, Mogao Grottoes, Dunhuang City, Gansu Province

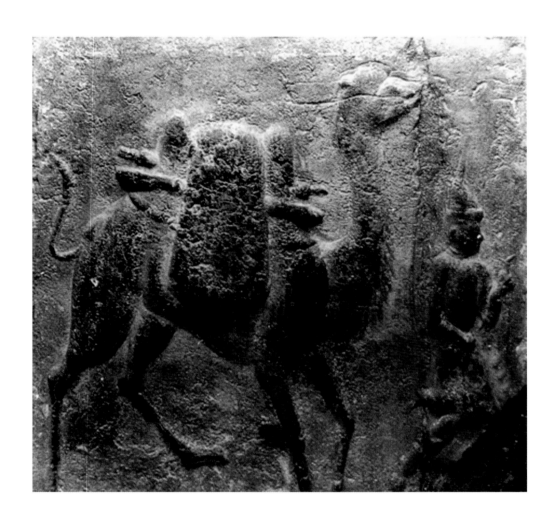

胡人引驼图

唐

砖刻

Brick Carving of Camel Leading by Hu Businessman

Tang Dynasty

Brick Carving

胡人着波斯装，一手执缰引驼，一手拄手杖
跋涉。骆驼长脖高扬，驮着货物跟随，反映
出当年丝绸之路上的贸易情景。唐代是"丝
绸之路"上贸易活动达到鼎盛的时期，中亚、
西亚、北非，以至地中海沿岸各国同唐王朝
往来频繁，同时也促进了医药学的交流。敦
煌佛爷庙唐墓出土。

敦煌市文化馆藏

The Hu businessman in this painting wears
Persian clothes. He is leading a camel in one
hand and walking with a cane in the other hand.
The camel carries the goods, keeping its head
high up. This painting reflects a scene of trade
on the Silk Road at that time. Trade activity
on the Silk Road was in a period of great
prosperity in the Tang Dynasty. Many countries
exchanged frequently with Tang, including
countries in the Central Asia, West Asia, North
Africa and countries along the Mediterranean
Sea. It promoted the exchange of medicine
and pharmacology at the same time. The brick
carving was unearthed in the Tang Tomb of
Buddha Temple in Dunhuang.
Preserved in Dunhuang Cultural Center

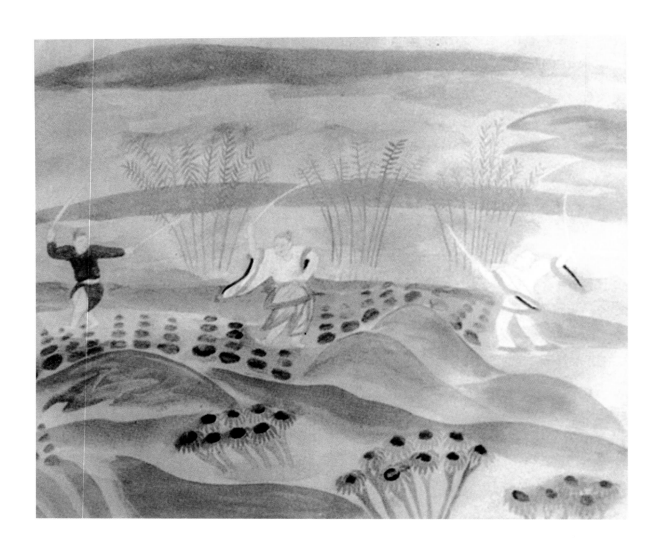

刀术壁画

五代

壁画

画面表现的是在一片旷野中，三位武士执刀

武练的情景。

甘肃敦煌莫高窟第 61 窟壁画

Fresco of Sabre Play

The Five Dynasties

Fresco

The painting shows that three warriors are
exercising with sabre in hand in the wilderness.
In Cave No. 61, Mogao Grottoes, Dunhuang
City, Gansu Province

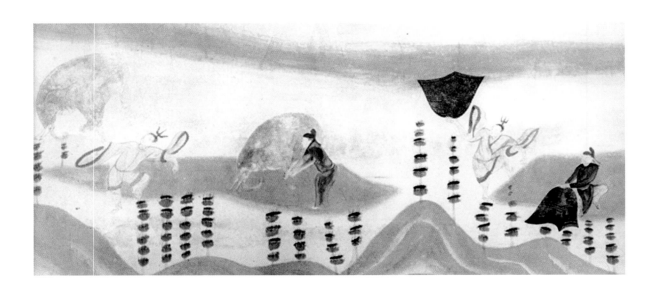

举象、擎钟壁画

五代

壁画

Fresco of Elephant and Bell Lifting

The Five Dynasties

Fresco

该壁画绘于窟内西壁，为佛教故事画之一节。图中左侧一人单臂将一只大象举起，中间一人双手执象腿正要上举；右侧第一人双手扶一大钟，似正在考虑如何将其举起，而第二人已将一口大钟擎起。图的背景为一片原野，使画面更具气势。

甘肃敦煌莫高窟第 61 窟壁画

The fresco is painted on the western wall of the cave and depicts a section of the Buddhist stories. On the left, one person is lifting an elephant with one arm while the man standing in the middle prepares to hold an elephant's legs. On the right, one man puts his hands on a big bell as if thinking how to lift it and the other man has lifted a big bell up. The picture is spectacular with a wild field as the background. In Cave No 61, Mogao Grottoes, Dunhuang City, Gansu Province

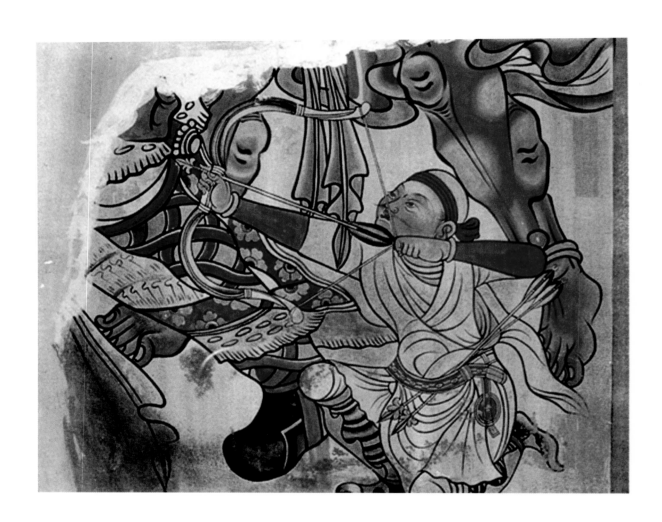

武士跪射图壁画

五代

壁画

Fresco of a Warrior Shooting on His Knee

The Five Dynasties

Fresco

画面中，一武士头戴枣红色巾，腰挂箭矢，左膝跪地，正弯弓向右侧上方的目标瞄准。由射手的装束看，画面表现的应是一位北方少数民族武士的形象。壁画绘于窟内南壁。

甘肃敦煌莫高窟第 346 窟壁画

In the painting, a warrior kneeling down on his left knee is drawing his bow at the target on the right upper side. He wears a purplish red head scarf with the arrows hanging on his waist. His clothing shows that he is a minority warrior in the north. This painting is on the southern wall of the grotto.

In Cave No. 346, Mogao Grottoes, Dunhuang City, Gansu Province

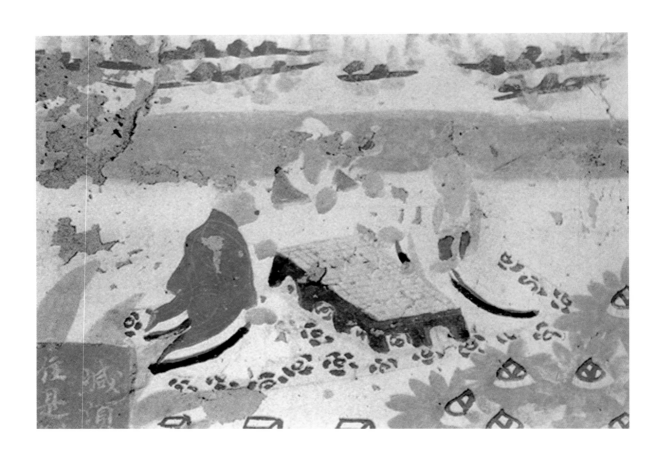

弈棋图壁画

五代

壁画

Fresco of Playing Weiqi

The Five Dynasties

Fresco

该图为窟中《维摩变》壁画的一部分，图中有一长方形的围棋盘，盘面棋局纹道较为清晰，棋盘两侧，各有一人，分别穿红、绿长袍，在静坐对弈。这幅画是对现实生活中弈棋活动的形象反映。

甘肃瓜州（原安西）县榆林窟第 30 窟壁画

It is a part of the frescoes of "Wei Mo Bian" (*Illustration of Vimalakirti Sutra*). In the painting, there is an oblong chessboard with clear tracks. Sitting silently on two sides of the board, two men， one in a red robe, the other in a green robe, are playing chess. This painting vividly depicts the chess playing activity in real life at that time.

In Cave No. 30, Yulin Grottoes, Guazhou County (Former Anxi County), Gansu Province

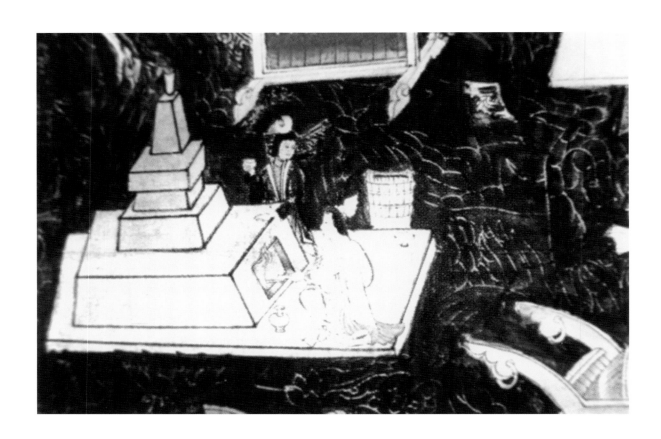

酿酒图

西夏

壁画

Fresco of Wine Making

Western Xia Dynasty

Fresco

该窟东壁南侧《千手千眼观音》壁画中对称地绘有两幅《酿酒图》。画面中央画一灶台，上安一套层叠覆压的方形器皿。一妇女于灶前执柴烧火，炉膛内火苗炽烈。左侧置一陶质酒壶。另一妇女于灶右，右手持钵。另置酒壶、木桶各一。有研究者认为这是我国最早的蒸酒形象资料。

甘肃瓜州（原安西）榆林窟西夏第 3 窟壁画

Two paintings of Wine Making are symmetrically placed in the Fresco of Thousand-hand and Thousand-eye Avalokitesvara on the south side of the eastern wall in this grotto. There is a hearth in the middle of the painting with a set of stack-up square-shaped vessels on it. A woman in front of the hearth is making a fiercely burning fire. There is a ceramic flagon on the left side of the hearth. On the right side, another woman is holding an earthen bowl in her right hand. Besides, there is another flagon and a wooden vat in this painting. According to some researchers, this is the earliest image of wine making in China.

In Cave No. 3, Yulin Grottoes, Guazhou County (former Anxi County), Gansu Province

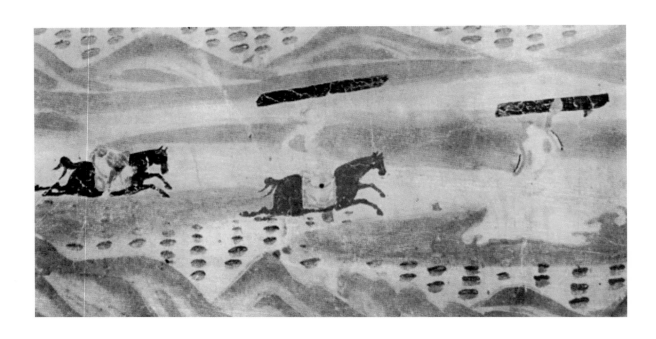

马术图壁画

宋
壁画

Fresco of Equestrianism

Song Dynasty

Fresco

此图绘于窟内西壁，表现的是佛教故事中须达拿太子和同伴们一起习武较力的故事。画面中三位骑者，自左向右疾驰。右一人立于象背上，居中者立于马上，二人均单手举一巨型横木；左边一人，坠于马侧俯身拾物，极为惊险。这是对现实生活中马术技巧的生动表现。

甘肃敦煌莫高窟第 61 窟壁画

This fresco is on the western wall of the grotto. The painting reproduces the story of Crown Prince Sudana and his companions practising martial arts described in the Buddhist tales. Three riders are galloping at full speed from the left to the right. The right rider is on an elephant and the middle rider is on a horse, both of whom are lifting heavy traverses. And the rider on the left is bending over from one side of the horse to pick up something, which is quite breath-taking. The painting vividly shows the equestrianism in the real life at that time.

In Cave No. 61, Mogao Grottoes, Dunhuang City, Gansu Province

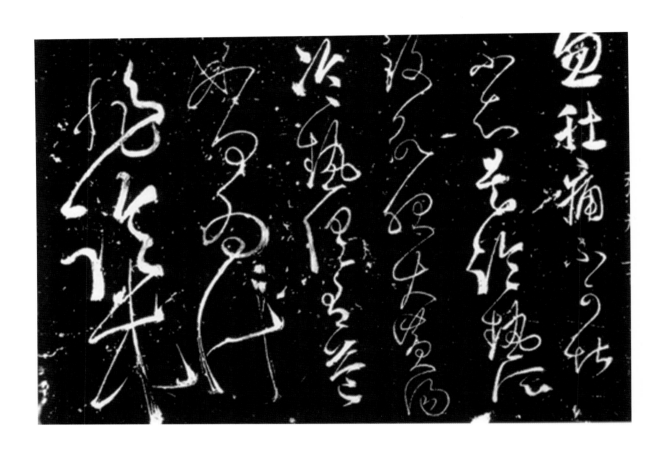

张旭肚痛贴刻石

宋

刻石

原图：纵 124 厘米，横 56 厘米

Stone Carving of Zhang Xu's "Du Tong Tie" Collywobbles Formula

Song Dynasty

Stone Carving

Original Painting: Width 124 cm/ Length 56 cm

刻石为竖形。两面分三截刻，共 48 行，每行 6 字。刻石正面为五代后梁时僧人彦修的草书刻石。草书内容为《寄边衣诗》及《入洛诗》。碑阴下方摹刻唐张旭《肚痛贴》30 字。释文为："忽肚痛不可堪，不知是冷热所致，取服大黄汤，冷热具有益，如何为计，非临床。"北宋嘉祐三年（1058）刻。

西安碑林博物馆藏

Carved into three parts on both sides of this vertical stone are 48 lines with 6 Chinese characters in each line. On the front of the stone is the engraving in cursive script of Yan Xiu, a monk in the Late Liang Dynasty of Five Dynasties. The contents of this engraving are two poems—"Ji Bian Yi Shi" and "Ru Luo Shi". There are 29 Chinese characters on the bottom of the back of the stone. It is the "Du Tong Tie" Collywobbles Formula by Zhang Xu of the Tang Dynasty, which means: "If you suddenly have an unbearable stomachache, whether it is caused by cold or heat, you can take the decoction of Chinese rhubarb. It works for whatever causes. This is non-clinical therapy." The stone was carved in the third year of the Jiayou Period of the Northern Song Dynasty (1058). Preserved in Xi'an Forest of Stone Steles Museum

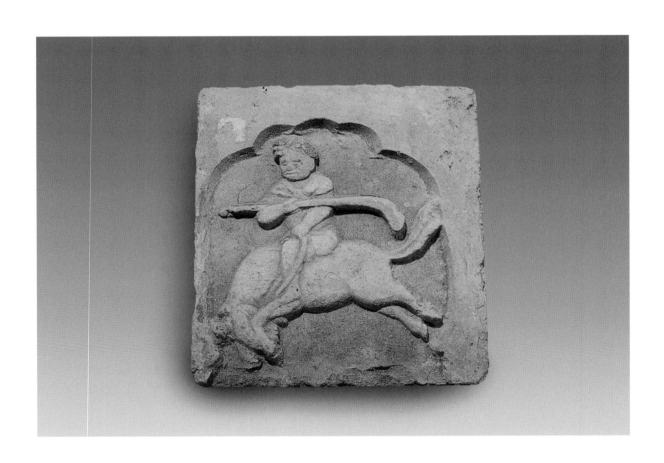

打马球画像砖

宋

画像砖

25 厘米 × 24 厘米 × 4.5 厘米

Embossed Brick with Polo Playing Portrait

Song Dynasty

Brick

25 cm × 24 cm × 4.5 cm

画像砖近于正方形。浮雕的画面上，骑于马上的击球手右手执球杖，左手勒缰，眼睛注视着前方。所骑之马，头抵向前蹄，后蹄撩起，尾巴上扬。整个画面表现了将要进入比赛的一刹那。

中国体育博物馆藏

This embossed brick is almost square in shape. On the surface, a batter on a horse is keeping his eyes forward. He is holding a ball rod in his right hand and drawing the rein with his left hand. The horse is pushing its head against its fore hoofs, holding up its hind hoofs and keeping its tail high up. It shows the moment of going to participate in a polo game.
Preserved in the China Sports Museum

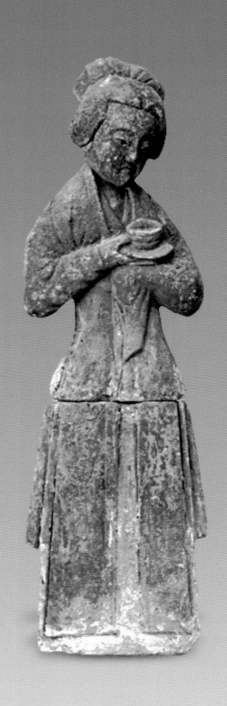

砖雕彩绘侍女俑

金

砖雕

高 57.5 厘米

砖雕线条简洁流畅，富有生活气息。

山西博物院藏

Colored Brick Carving of a Terracotta Maidservant

Jin Dynasty

Brick Carving

Height 57.5 cm

This artwork has succinct lines and is imbued with vitality.

Preserved in Shanxi Museum

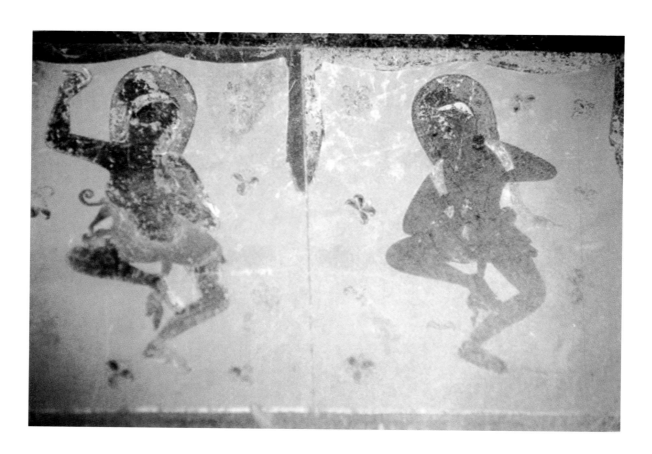

欢喜金刚图

元
壁画

Fresco of Delighted Vajra-bodhisattva

Yuan Dynasty

Fresco

藏传佛教密宗有一种以两性性接触为途径的
特殊修禅法，称为"欲乐定"或"双身法"，
与今之气功与性事养生均不无联系。符合修
此禅法的异性称为"欢喜金刚"或"手印"等。
图示即双方在性接触前之嬉戏舞姿。

甘肃敦煌莫高窟第 465 窟壁画

In Tibetan Esoteric Buddhism, there is a special
meditation method by bisexual contact which
is called Yuleding or Shuangshenfa. It is related
to qigong and sexual health care. People of
different sexes studying this Zen method are
all called the Delighted Vajra-bodhisattva or
Handprint. The painting shows the foreplay
dancing before their sexual contact.
In Cave No. 465, Mogao Grottoes, Dunhuang
City, Gansu Province

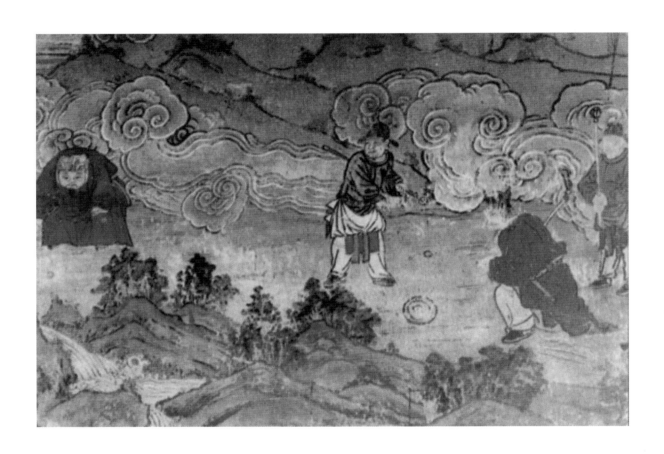

捶丸图壁画

元

壁画

纵 112 厘米，横 175 厘米

Fresco of Batting

Yuan Dynasty

Fresco

Width 112 cm/ Length 175 cm

捶丸图绘于明应王殿西壁北部的上层。在深山之巅有一块平地,两位身着米色袍的官吏,分置东西,持棒攻球。官吏身后各有一年轻侍者持铜锤侍立。画面上山势起伏,溪流蜿蜒而过,树木长于山侧,呈现出优美的自然风光。

山西省洪洞县广胜寺水神庙明应王殿壁画

This painting is on the northern upper part of the western wall in King Mingying's Hall. Two government officials in cream-coloured robes are standing on a piece of flat land on the top of a high mountain. Opposing each other in the east and the west, they are batting with ball rods. A young servant is holding a copper hammer behind each of them. With the mountains being high or low, the ravine stream meandering, and the trees growing on the versant, the natural scenery is quite graceful.

In King Mingying's Hall of Guangsheng Water God Temple, Hongdong County, Shanxi Province

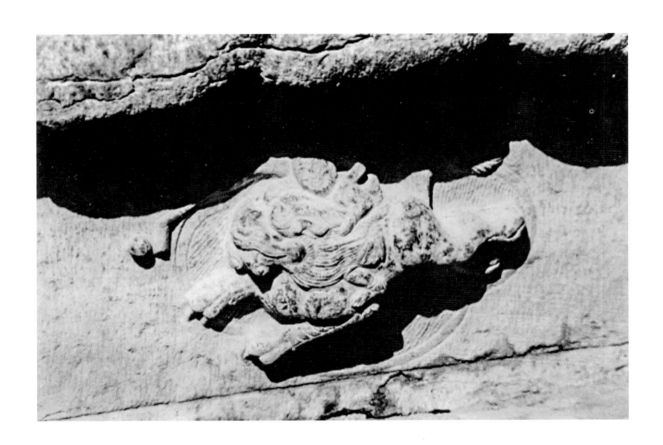

骑狮击球图

元

石雕

Embossment of Batting on Lion

Yuan Dynasty

Stone Carving

山东省济南市长清区灵岩寺墓塔石雕。画面采用浮雕的形式，刻画了一骑狮人举杖击球的情形。图中的雄师四蹄腾空，翘首扬尾，做飞奔之状；骑狮者手执球杖，俯身击打前面的小球。

山东省济南市长清区灵岩寺藏

The stone embrossment sits in Lingyan Temple of Changqing Districe, Jinan City, Shandong Province. This embossed engraving describes a player batting on a lion. In the picture, the lion is running at full speed with its hoofs rising high into the air, its head high up and its tail raised. Meanwhile, the rider is bending over to bat the small ball in the front.

Preserved in Lingyan Temple, Changqing District, Jinan City, Shandong Province

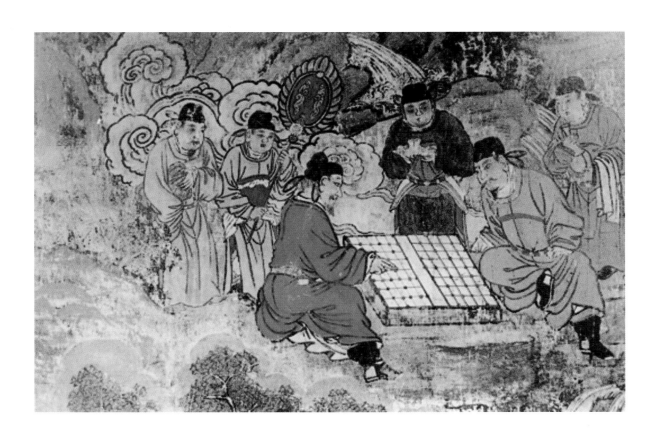

对局图壁画

元
壁画
纵 97 厘米，横 152 厘米

Fresco of Chess Playing

Yuan Dynasty

Fresco

Height 97 cm/ Length 152 cm

图中倚石席地对坐攻棋者二人，左边一人目光炯炯，右手举棋未定，右边一人聚精会神地注视着对方的攻势。他们身后各立二位侍者观战。棋局中间画有一河界，纵线九条亦同于象棋，唯横线比象棋多一条。但从整个棋局看，应为一种象棋局势。

山西省洪洞县广胜寺水神庙明应王殿壁画

In the fresco, two players are leaning on stones and sitting face to face on the ground. The eagle-eyed player on the left is holding an uncertain chessman in his right hand, while the player on the right is attentively watching his opponent's offensive action. Behind each player, two attendants are watching the game. A river is painted in the middle of the chessboard and nine vertical lines are also drawn there, which shows that this is almost the same as the Chinese chess we have now. But it has one more horizontal line than Chinese chess. However, from the whole composition, it can be inferred that this actually is a kind of Chinese chess game.
In King Mingying's Hall of Guangsheng Water God Temple, Hongdong County, Shanxi Province

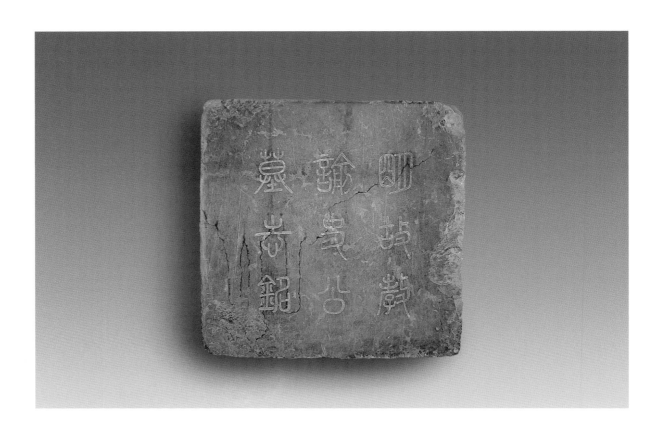

明故教谕史公墓志盖

明

石质

61 厘米 ×61 厘米 ×10.5 厘米

Tombstone of Revered Late Ming Dynasty Education Instructor Mr. Shi

Ming Dynasty

Stone

61 cm × 61 cm × 10.5 cm

该墓志盖为正方形。上有明·翰林修撰吕柟
篆书"明故教谕史公墓志铭"字样。陪葬品。
保存基本完整。陕西省征集。

陕西医史博物馆藏

This square tombstone was inscribed with
words in seal script written by Lu Nan, an
Imperial Academy Senior Officer in the Ming
Dynasty, meaning "epitaph of the revered late
Ming Dynasty Education Instructor Mr. Shi".
This burial object was collected in Shaanxi
Province and is still in good shape.

Preserved in Shaanxi Museum of Medical History

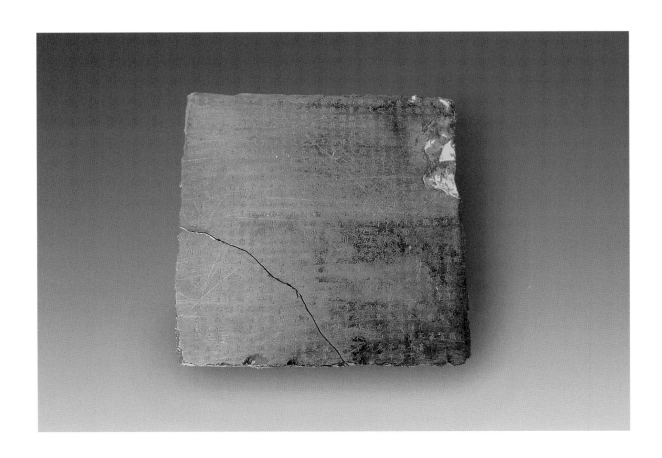

明故教谕史公墓志铭

明

石质

61 厘米 ×61 厘米 ×10.5 厘米

Tombstone of Revered Late Ming Dynasty Education Instructor Mr. Shi

Ming Dynasty

Stone

61 cm×61 cm×10.5 cm

该墓志铭为正方形。墓志铭为明代进士·翰林院检讨、文学家及医家王九思撰文。志为楷书，共 700 余字，介绍高平教谕史章、字文焕的生平及去世原因等。陪葬品。稍残。陕西省征集。

陕西医史博物馆藏

This square tombstone was carved with an epitaph of more than 700 Chinese characters in regular script written by Wang Jiusi, a Ming Dynasty Imperial Scholar, Imperial Academy Editor of History, man of letters and doctor. The epitaph presents the life experience and cause of death of a late Education Instructor of Gaoping County by the name of Shi Zhang (styled Shi Wenhuan). This burial object was collected in Shaanxi Province and was slightly damaged. Preserved in Shaanxi Museum of Medical History

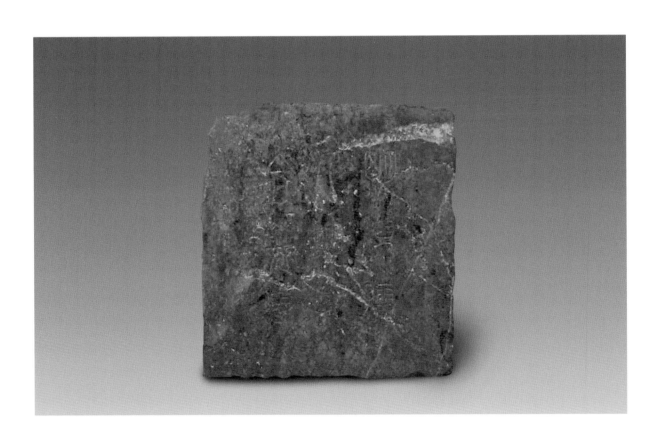

倪儒人陶氏合葬墓石刻

明

石质

54.7 厘米 ×56.3 厘米 ×10.8 厘米

Tombstone of Scholar Ni and His Wife Tao's Joint Tomb

Ming Dynasty

Stone

54.7 cm × 56.3 cm × 10.8 cm

碑刻为长方形。该石刻在上海南汇发现，与"明倪儒人陶氏合葬墓墓志铭文石刻"是一整体。一为篆刻大字"明倪儒人陶氏合葬墓石刻"，一为楷书小字墓志铭内容。据专家考证内有针刺治疗白内障的记载，前后均为明代江南四大才子之一文徵明晚年珍迹。倪儒人详情待考。该藏为大字碑刻。碑刻表面损坏较严重，多处字迹模糊不清。

中华医学会 / 上海中医药大学医史博物馆藏

This rectangular tombstone was found in Nanhui District, Shanghai. This picture and the next one entitled "Tombstone of Scholar Ni and His Hife Tao's Joint Tomb" are the photos of the two parts of the same tombstone. On the front side of this tombstone are inscribed words in big seal script meaning "Tombstone Inscription of Scholar Ni and His Wife Tao's Joint Tomb" and on the back of the tombstone is inscribed the epigraph in small regular script in which there are, according to the experts, descriptions about acupuncture treatment of cataract. Both of the carvings were written by Wen Zhengming, one of the Four Gifted Scholars in south China in the Ming Dynasty, in his later years. However, the information about Scholar Ni remains to be studied. This picture is about the side written with big characters. Since the surface of the tombstone has been seriously damaged, many characters are too vague to be identified.
Preserved in Chinese Medical Association/Museum of Chinese Medicine, Shanghai University of Traditional Chinese Medicine

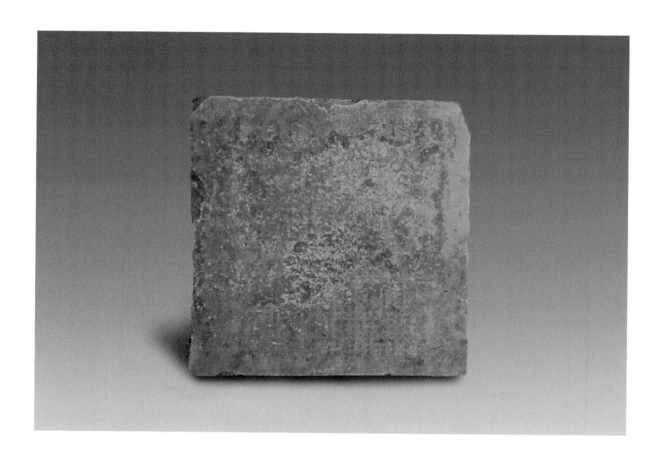

明倪儒人陶氏合葬墓墓志铭文石刻

明

石质

56.2 厘米 × 56.8 厘米 × 10.5 厘米

Tombstone of Scholar Ni and His Wife Tao's Joint Tomb

Ming Dynasty

Stone

56.2 cm × 56.8 cm × 10.5 cm

碑刻为长方形。该石刻在上海南汇发现，与"明倪儒人陶氏合葬墓石刻"是一整体。一为篆刻大字"明倪儒人陶氏合葬墓石刻"，一为楷书小字墓志铭内容。据专家考证内有针刺治疗白内障的记载，前后均为明代江南四大才子之一文徵明晚年珍迹。倪儒人详情待考。该藏为小字铭文部分碑刻。碑刻表面损坏较严重，多处字迹模糊不清。

中华医学会／上海中医药大学医史博物馆藏

This rectangular carved tombstone was found in Nanhui District, Shanghai. This picture and the previous one entitled "Tombstone of Scholar Ni and His Wife Tao's Joint Tomb" are the photos of the two sides of the same tombstone. On the front side of this tombstone are inscribed words meaning "Tombstone Inscription of Scholar Ni and His Wife Tao's Joint Tomb" and on the back of the tombstone is inscribed the epigraph in small regular script in which there are, according to the experts, descriptions about acupuncture treatment of cataract. Both of the carvings were written by Wen Zhengming, one of the Four Gifted Scholars in south China in the Ming Dynasty, in his later years. However, the information about Scholar Ni remains to be studied. This picture is about the side written with small regular script. Since the surface of the tombstone has been seriously damaged, many characters are too vague to be identified. Preserved in Chinese Medical Association/Museum of Chinese Medicine, Shanghai University of Traditional Chinese Medicine

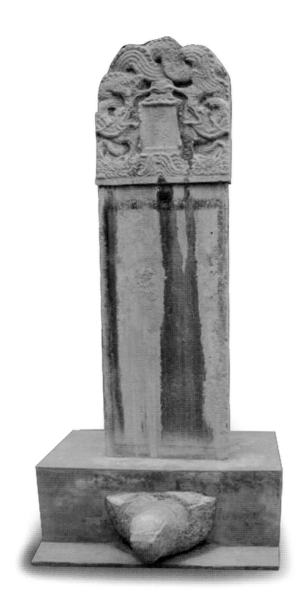

重修武子望家祠碑

明

石质

252 厘米 ×81 厘米 ×23.5 厘米

**Tablet Inscribed with Records of
Rebuilding Wu Ziwang's Family
Ancestral Hall**

Ming Dynasty

Stone

252 cm × 81 cm × 23.5 cm

碑头为二龙戏珠石雕，内容主要为武子望家
祠修建情况及武氏的身世介绍。医药碑刻。
有残损。陕西省临潼区征集。

陕西医史博物馆藏

The head of the tablet is carved into a shape
of two dragons playing with a pearl. The main
contents on the stone are about Wu Ziwang's
life experience and the building of his family's
ancestral hall. It belongs to the category of
medical inscription. It was collected in Lintong
District, Shaanxi Province and has been
damaged.

Preserved in Shaanxi Museum of Medical History

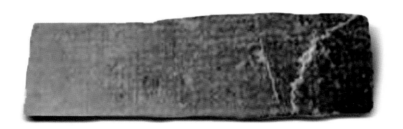

兴平药方碑

明清时期

石质

一石碑长 112 厘米，宽 33.5 厘米，厚 16 厘米

另一石碑长 100 厘米，宽 33.5 厘米，厚 16 厘米

Xingping Stone Tablets of Prescriptions

Ming or Qing Dynasty

Stone

One: Length 112 cm/ Width 33.5 cm/ Thickness 16 cm

The Other: Length 100 cm/ Width 33.5 cm/ Thickness 16 cm

药方碑，两件。陕西省兴平市桑镇征集。

陕西医史博物馆收藏

These two prescription stone tablets were collected in Sangzhen Town, Xingping City, Shaanxi Province.

Preserved in Shaanxi Museum of Medical History

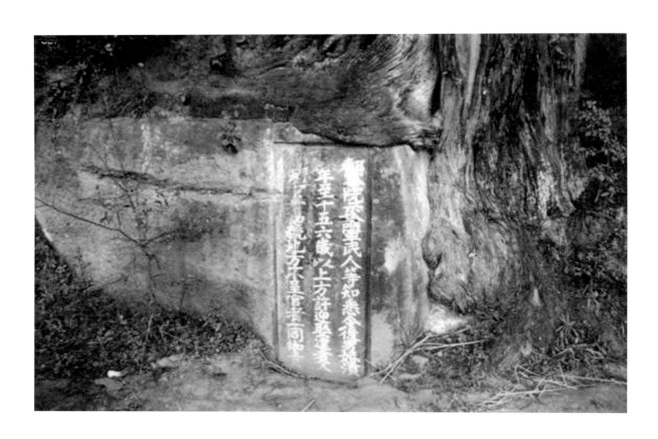

禁止早婚告示石刻

明

石刻

纵 140 厘米，横 23 厘米

Stone Inscription of "No Early Marriage" Announcement

Ming Dynasty

Stone

Width 140 cm/ Length 23 cm

正书阴刻，四行："都察院示谕军民人等知

悉，今后男婚须年至十五六岁以上方许迎娶，

违者父母重则枷，地方不呈官者，一同枷责。"

落款为大明万历十三年 (1585)。石刻位于四

川省广元市剑阁县的古驿道上，距剑阁县城

15 千米的龙源镇以北 1 千米处。保存完好。

四川省广元市剑阁县古驿

The stone was incised in regular script in intaglio in four lines with the announcement meaning "it is notified by the Court of Censors that all men should be above fifteen or sixteen years old when they get married. Any offender's parents will be put on cangues. If the local officials fail to report any offenders, they will be put on cangues too. " And the date is "Da Ming Wan Li Shi San Nian (the thirteenth year of Wanli Period of the Ming Dynasty) (1585)". The stone is located at a place on the former courier route 1 km to the north of Longyuan Town, which is 15 km away from Jiange County, Guangyuan City, Sichuan Province. Now the stone is still in good condition.

Jiange County, Guangyuan City, Sichuan Province

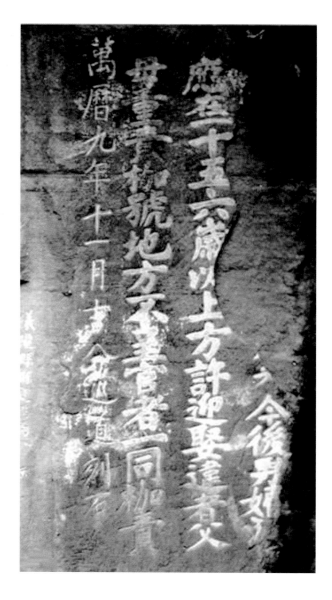

禁止早婚告示石刻

明

石刻

纵 165 厘米，横 80 厘米

Stone Inscription of "No Early Marriage" Announcement

Ming Dynasty

Stone

Width 165 cm/ Length 80 cm

石刻位于四川省仪陇县双盘乡凌云寨下高石坎村"十大碗"的一块名叫衬腰石的大岩石上。阴刻，正文3行楷书。第1行已剥蚀11字，经查考为"都察院示谕军民人等知悉"。落款为万历九年(1581)十一月吉分巡道(川北道保宁分巡道)刻石。

四川省仪陇县双盘乡凌云寨

The inscription is carved on a big rock named Chenyao Rock, which is located in Shi Da Wan in Lower Gaoshikan Village, Lingyun Zhai, Shuangpan Town, Yilong County, Sichuan Province. All Chinese characters on this rock were incised in intaglio, among which the main contents were inscribed in regular script in three lines. But the eleven characters in the first line have been corroded, which, after investigation, are believed to be "Du Cha Yuan Shi Yu Jun Min Ren Deng Xi Zhi", meaning "it is notified by the Court of Censors to all people". Below that is the inscription in Chinese characters "Wan Li Jiu Nian Shi Yi Yue Ji Fen Xun Dao Ke Shi", meaning "incised in the eleventh month of the ninth year of Wanli Period (1581) by the Censor of Baoning District under the Administration of the Northern Sichuan Prefecture".

Lingyun Zhai, Shuangpan Town, Yilong County, Sichuan Province

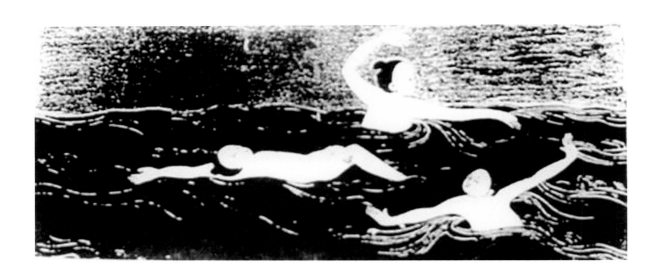

游泳图壁画

明
壁画

Mural of Swimming

Ming Dynasty
Mural

画面中河水荡漾，三位头挽发髻的裸体习水
者，正在畅游。其姿态优美，生动活泼。

西藏自治区日喀则市扎什伦布寺壁画

In the mural, three naked swimmers with their
hair coiled into buns are gracefully and lively
swimming in the rippling river.

Mural in Tashilhunpo Monastery, Shigatse City,

Tibet Autonomous Region

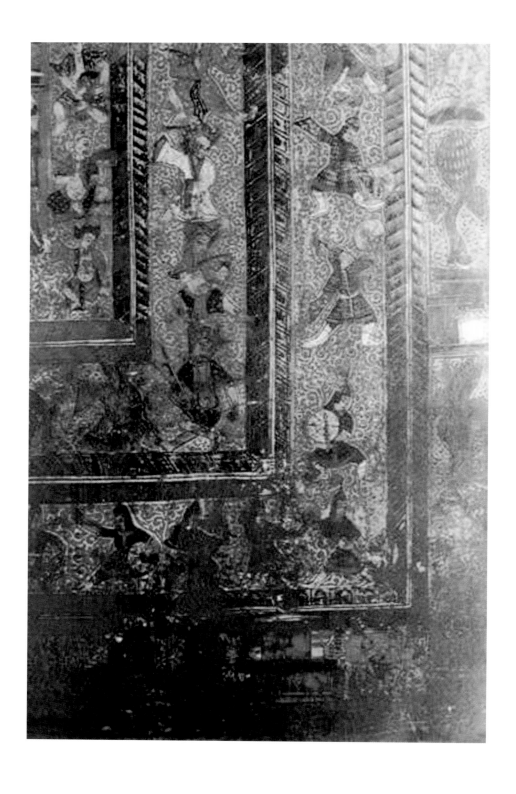

演武图壁画

明

壁画

此图位于殿东壁北侧，为《毗沙门天图》的右下角部分。画面共分四重，其中第二、三、四重皆为执各种兵器的武士和各路天神。众武士、天神或挽盾防护，或挥剑击砍，姿态各异。依《藏刀十三式》载，藏族刀法中就有"龙出西海"、"鹰旋雪岭"、"马驰平原"、"豹跃深涧"等术式，此图所展示的正是武士们依据藏族拳法、刀法，在一招一式地演武。

西藏自治区古格都城寺院大威德殿壁画

Mural of Tibetan Martial Arts Practicing

Ming Dynasty

Mural

The mural, located at the northern side of the eastern wall in the Guge Kingdom Temple, is the lower right part of the "Pi Sha Men Tian Tu Picture". It is divided into four levels, among which level two, level three and level four are carved with warriors and gods holding various weapons in their hands. Some of them are wielding their swords to attack and the others are defending with shields. According to the book "Zang Dao Shi San Shi" (*Thirteen Models of Exercising the Tibetan Knife*), there are many Tibetan martial arts knife styles such as "dragon leaping out of the west sea", "eagle circling over the snow-clad mountain", "horse galloping on the plain" and "leopard jumping over the deep gully". And this picture just shows how warriors are practicing Tibetan martial arts knives in accordance with the book.

Mural in Yamantaka Hall of the Guge Kingdom Temple, Tibet Autonomous Region

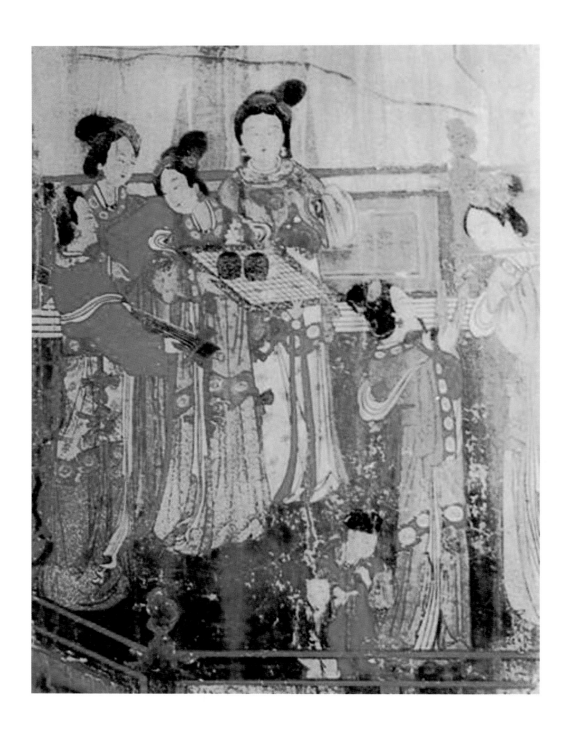

侍女围棋图壁画

明

壁画

纵 126 厘米，横 94 厘米

壁画绘于圣母殿北壁西部。图中的侍女吹着横笛和笙，捧着围棋、金盏、奁盒和古琴，供圣母享用。侍女手中的围棋局和棋盘、装棋子的围棋盒，清晰可见。

山西省汾阳市圣母庙圣母殿壁画

Mural of Maidservants and Weiqi

Ming Dynasty

Mural

Width 126 cm/ Length 94 cm

The mural is located at the western side of the northern wall in the Goddess Temple. In this mural, some maidservants are blowing fife and sheng instruments; the others are holding weiqi, a gold cup, a toilet case and a guqin instrument respectively in their hands for the Goddess to use. The weiqi board and box held in the hands of the maidservant can be clearly distinguished in the mural.

Mural in the Goddess Hall of the Goddess Temple, Fenyang City, Shanxi Province

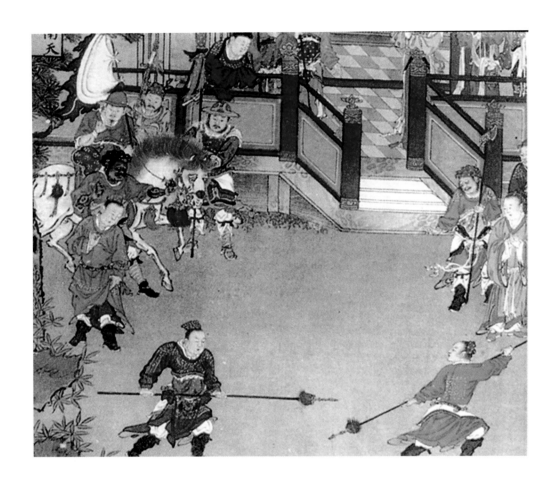

太子共南天国斗武艺图壁画摹本

明

纵 37 厘米，横 51 厘米

Tracing of Fresco of Crown Prince Fighting with Warriors from Southern Kingdom

Ming Dynasty

Width 37 cm/ Length 51 cm

原壁画已于清代毁于火灾，此为明代匠师的
摹本《释迦世尊应化示迹图》之一，描述的
是佛传故事画之一节。图中，太子与南天国
武士正在比试枪术武艺。

山西省太原市崇善寺大雄宝殿两掖长廊壁画

The original mural was destroyed by fire in the
Qing Dynasty. This is one of the exact copies
of *Pictures of Sakyamuni's Life and Teaching*
by craftsman in the Ming Dynasty. It is about
Buddhist stories. In the mural, the Crown Prince
is contesting with warriors from Southern
Kingdom.

Along the corridors of the main hall in Chongshan
Temple, Taiyuan City, Shanxi Province

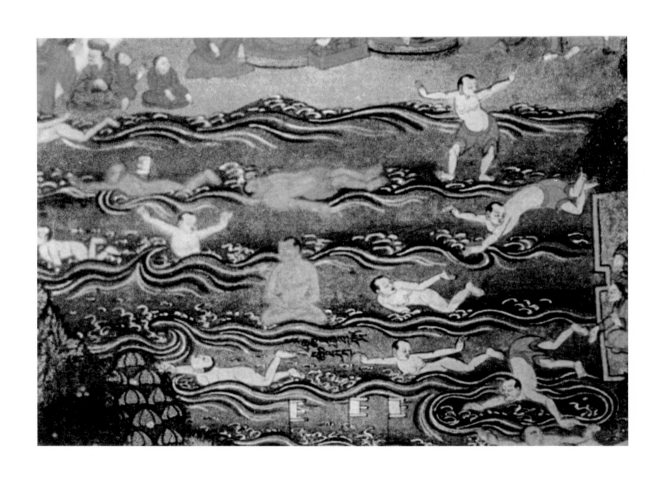

游泳图壁画

清

壁画

Mural of Swimming

Qing Dynasty

Mural

在一波涛涌起的江水中，一群喜泳者正在击水竞游。画面将游泳者击水、浮水和跳水的各种姿态描绘得活泼生动，形象逼真。

西藏自治区拉萨市布达拉宫壁画

A group of swimmers are splashing and competing in a wavy river. The image of how swimmers are splashing, floating and diving is really true to life.

In the Potala Palace, Lhasa City, Tibet Autonomous Region

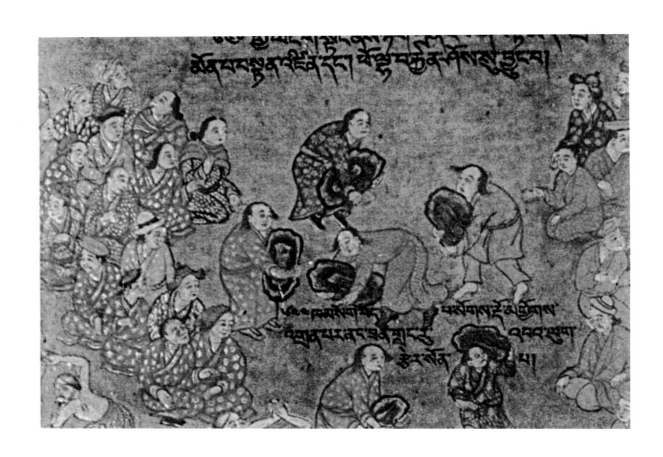

布达拉宫落成仪式图局部

清

壁画

原图：纵 40 厘米，横 31 厘米

Part of the Mural of Potala Palace Inauguration Ceremony

Qing Dynasty

Mural

Original Painting: Width 40 cm/ Length 31 cm

这是表现为庆祝红宫落成典礼而举行仪式的一幅壁画的局部——举石竞力图。举石，是古代体育活动中举重项目的形式之一，画面中表现了六位力士，在观众围成的场地内，做抱石、举石和扛石的练力比赛，这是对当时举重活动的形象描绘。

西藏自治区拉萨市布达拉宫西大殿二楼画廊壁画

This part of the mural about celebrating the Red Palace Inauguration Ceremony is called Picture of Stone Lifting Competition. Stone lifting was one of the sports forms of weight-lifting in ancient times. In the mural, surrounded by the spectators, six competitors are holding, lifting or shouldering stones. The weight-lifting image is vividly portrayed in the mural.

In the gallery on the second floor of the Great West Hall of the Potala Palace, Lhasa City, Tibet Autonomous Region

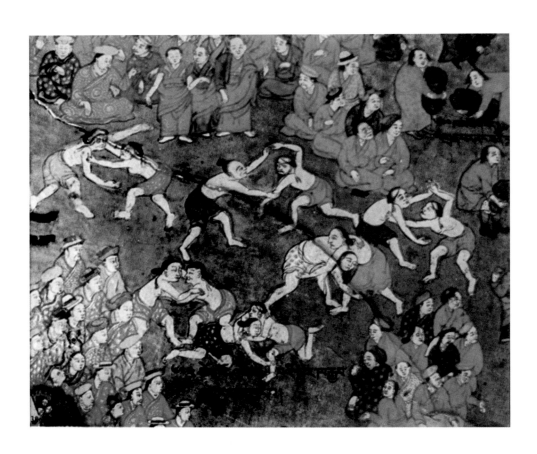

布达拉宫落成仪式图局部

清

壁画

原壁画：纵 40 厘米，横 31 厘米

Part of the Mural of Potala Palace Inauguration Ceremony

Qing Dynasty

Mural

Original Painting: Width 40 cm / Length 31 cm

这是表现为庆祝红宫落成典礼而举行仪式的一幅壁画的局部。图中，六对摔跤手正在进行激烈的摔跤竞赛，这些摔跤手均上身赤裸，下着短裤，表现出奋力竞争的态势，周围坐有观看比赛的喇嘛。

西藏自治区拉萨市布达拉宫西大殿二楼画廊壁画

In this part of the mural about celebrating the Red Palace Inauguration Ceremony, six wrestlers dressed in shorts only are sparing no efforts to compete, and some lamas are sitting around and watching the game.

In the gallery on the second floor of the Great West Hall of the Potala Palace, Lhasa City, Tibet Autonomous Region

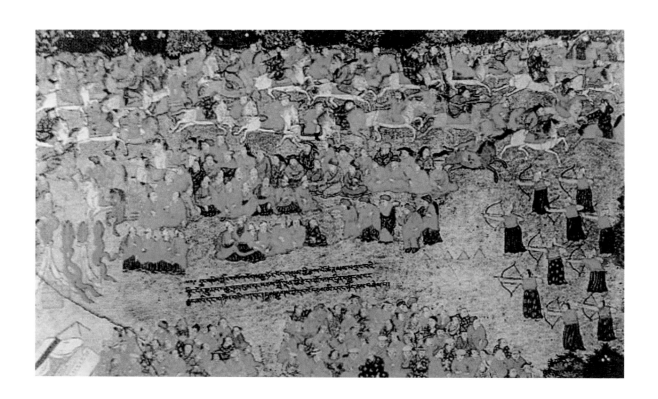

布达拉宫落成仪式图局部

清

壁画

原图：纵 40 厘米，横 31 厘米

Part of the Mural of Potala Palace Inauguration Ceremony

Qing Dynasty

Mural

Original Painting: Width 40 cm/ Length 31 cm

这是表现为庆祝红宫落成典礼而举行仪式的一幅壁画的局部。画面中，有数位头戴藏帽、身穿红绿长袍的射手们执弓对靶而射。整个画面展现出一派热烈的竞赛气氛。

西藏自治区拉萨市布达拉宫西大殿二楼画廊壁画

In this part of the mural about celebrating the Red Palace Inauguration Ceremony, several shooters in traditional Tibetan hats and red or green robes are shooting at the targets with their bows. The whole picture presents a warm atmosphere of competition.

In the gallery on the second floor of the Great West Hall of the Potala Palace, Lhasa City, Tibet Autonomous Region

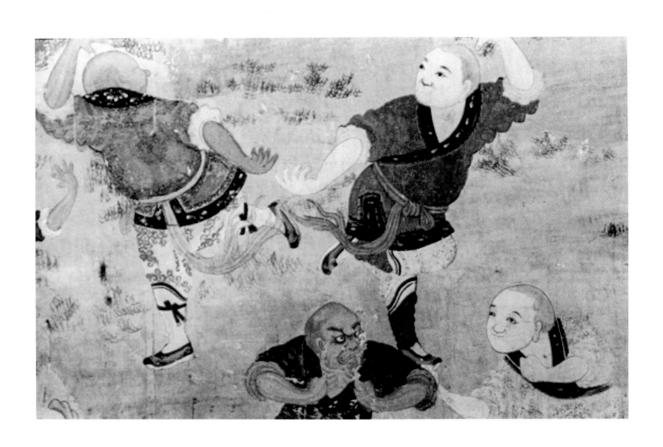

拳术演练图壁画

清

壁画

Mural of Chinese Boxing Practice

Qing Dynasty

Mural

白衣殿壁画描绘的是少林寺和尚演武和初唐少林寺十三棍僧救唐王的故事内容。此图是白衣殿壁画的局部，表现了少林寺僧演练拳术的情景。

河南市登封市少林寺白衣殿壁画

The murals in the White Clothing Hall portray the scene of martial arts practice of the monks in the Shaolin Temple and the story about the 13 Shaolin Stick-monks rescuing the King of Tang in the Early Tang Dynasty. This is just a part of the murals in the White Clothing Hall which describes how the monks in Shaolin Temple practice martial arts.

In the White Clothing Hall of Shaolin Temple, Dengfeng City, Henan Province

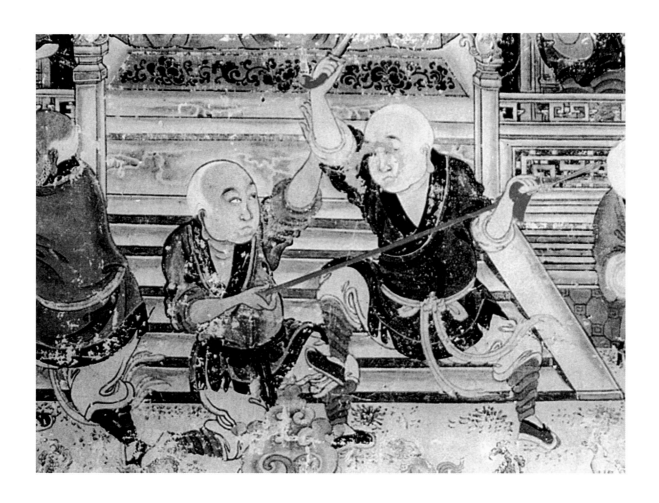

器械演练图壁画

清
壁画

Mural of Martial Arts Practice with Weapons

Qing Dynasty

Mural

此图为白衣殿壁画的局部，反映的是少林寺
僧持器械技击演练的场面，生动地再现了古
代少林武术的威武场面。

河南省登封市少林寺白衣殿壁画

This is just a part of the murals in the White
Clothing Hall of the Shaolin Temple, which
describes how the monks in Shaolin Temple
practice martial arts with weapons. It vividly
reproduces the magnificent and mighty scene of
martial arts practice in ancient Shaolin Temple.
In the White Clothing Hall of Shaolin Temple,
Dengfeng City, Henan Province

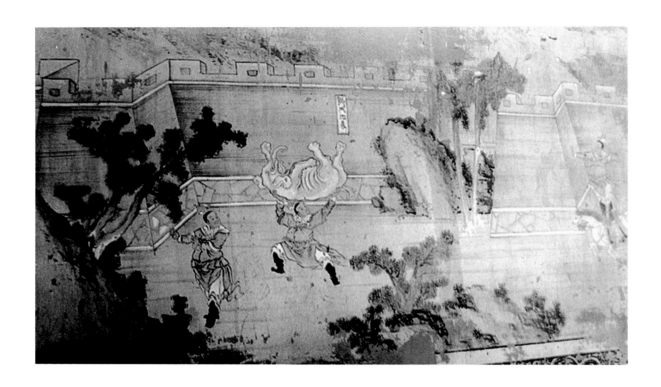

隔城抛象图壁画

清

纵 100 厘米，横 175 厘米

Fresco of Casting an Elephant from the City

Qing Dynasty

Width 100 cm/ Length 175 cm

该壁画绘于寺内三佛殿东壁北部，为释迦太子事迹之一。画面上地势广大，树木、山石、城墙及墙上垛口清晰可辨，太子正在抛举大象。图中人物像高约 25~30 厘米。

山西省太谷县净信寺壁画

The mural is painted on the northern part of the eastern wall of Three Buddhas Hall of the temple. It is about one of the stories of Crown Prince Sakyamuni. In this picture, trees, rocks, city walls and crenels are clear and distinguishable against the vast landscape. The Crown Prince is casting an elephant. Humans in the mural are about 25 to 30 cm high.

In Jingxin Temple, Taigu County, Shanxi Province

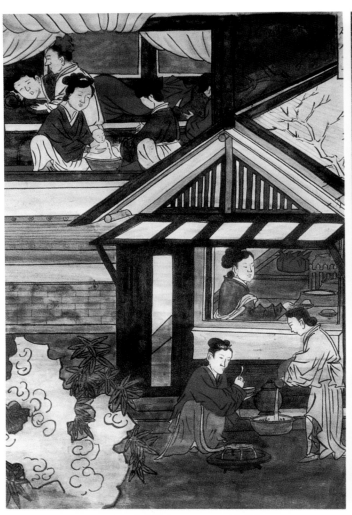

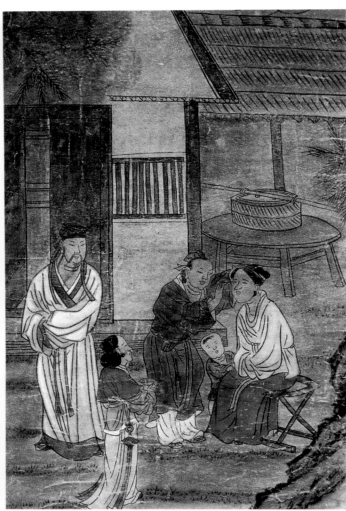

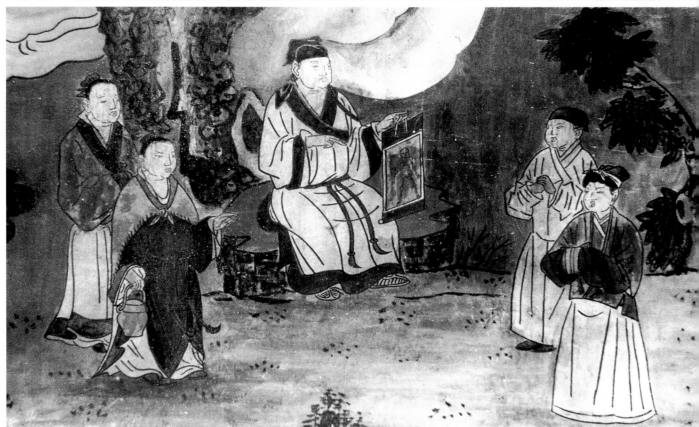

永乐宫壁画的医学内容（摹本）

永乐宫位于山西省芮城县永乐镇，是元代统治者替传为神仙的吕洞宾建的供奉庙观。在其纯阳殿和重阳殿的壁画中，有部分医药卫生的内容，上图左为洗儿图，上图右为点眼图，下图为骨骼图。

陕西医史博物馆藏

Mural (Facsimile) of Medicine Contents in Yongle Taoist Temple

Yongle Taoist Temple, located in Yongle Town, Ruicheng County, Shanxi Province, was built by the Yuan Dynasty government under an imperial decree for a Taoist Immortal by the name of Lü Dongbin. Some murals in the Chunyang Hall and Chongyang Hall in the temple are about medicine and health. The upper left picture is about washing a baby; the upper right one is about giving eye drops; and the bottom one is a picture of the human skeleton.

Preserved in Shaanxi Museum of Medical History

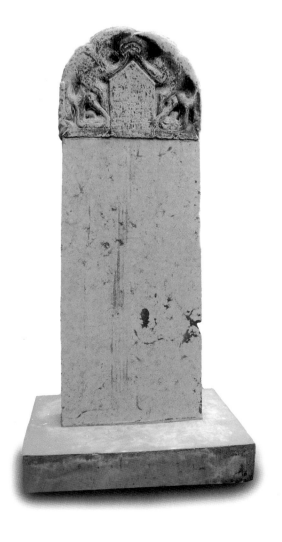

大秦景教流行中国碑

近现代

石质

宽 100 厘米，厚 26 厘米，通高 290
厘米

Nestorian Tablet

Modern Times

Stone

Width 100 cm/ Thickness 26 cm/

Height 290 cm

原碑为唐朝制作，存于陕西西安碑林博物馆。该碑介绍景教在中国的传播情况，其中有关于医学的内容。医药碑刻。完整无损。陕西医史博物馆复制。

陕西医史博物馆藏

The original tablet is in Xi'an Forest of Stone Steles Museum of Shaanxi Province. The inscription is about the spreading of Nestorianism in China and also about medicine. So this is also called a tablet of medicine. It is a replica made by Shaanxi Museum of Medical History and is still in good shape.

Preserved in Shaanxi Museum of Medical History

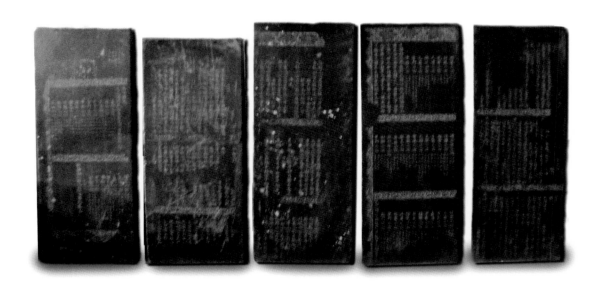

宋针灸铜人俞穴图经

近现代

石质

宽 46.8 厘米，厚 6.8 厘米，高 108~115 厘米

Stone Tablets with Song Dynasty's Diagram of Acupuncture Points

Modern Times

Stone

Width 46.8 cm/ Thickness 6.8 cm/ Height 108–115 cm

石碑呈长方形，上书宋王惟一《针灸铜人俞穴图经》的部分内容。医药碑刻。完整无损。此碑据宋代刻石残块复制。

陕西医史博物馆藏

These rectangular tablets present part of the contents of "Zhen Jiu Tong Ren Shu Xue Tu Jing"(*Illustrated Manual of Acupuncture Points of the Bronze Figure*) written by Wang Weiyi in the Song Dynasty. So these are also tablets of medicine. They are replicas of the damaged tablets of the Song Dynasty and are in good shape.

Preserved in Shaanxi Museum of Medical History

历代名医神碑

近现代

石质

宽 72 厘米，厚 9.5 厘米，高 159 厘米

Stone Tablet of Famous Doctors of All the Dynasties

Modern Times

Stone

Width 72 cm/ Thickness 9.5 cm/ Height 159 cm

碑头为半圆形，一碑两面，正面为孙真人风药论，背面为《历代名医神碑》的内容。医药碑刻。完整无损。原碑为明代，此为陕西省医史博物馆复制。

陕西医史博物馆藏

The tablet has a semicircular top. Words are inscribed on both sides. The front side is inscribed with Sun Simiao's analysis of rheumatism and its medicines, while the back side is inscribed with the contents of *Tablet of Famous Doctors of All the Dynasties*. So it is a tablet of medicine. It is a replica made by Shaanxi Museum of Medical History after the original tablets of the Ming Dynasty and is still in good shape.

Preserved in Shaanxi Museum of Medical History

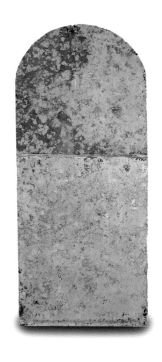

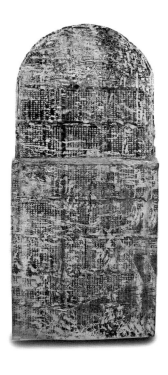

千金宝要碑

近现代

石质

宽 97 厘米，厚 17 厘米，高 227 厘米

碑头为半圆形，四通八面，楷书，内容主要为选录《千金要方》及部分验方共 900 余首。医药碑刻。有残。原碑为明代，此为陕西医史博物馆复制。

陕西医史博物馆藏

Stone Tablets of A Thousand Invaluable Prescriptions

Modern Times

Stone

Width 97 cm/ Thickness 17 cm/ Height 227 cm

These tablets have semicircular tops. On the eight sides of these four tablets are inscribed in regular script the selected prescriptions from the book "Qian Jin Yao Fang" (A Thousand Invaluable Prescriptions) and other proved prescriptions in a total of more than 900. So they are tablets of medicine. They are replicas made by Shaanxi Museum of Medical History after the original tablets of the Ming Dynsty and some of them have been damaged.

Preserved in Shaanxi Museum of Medical History

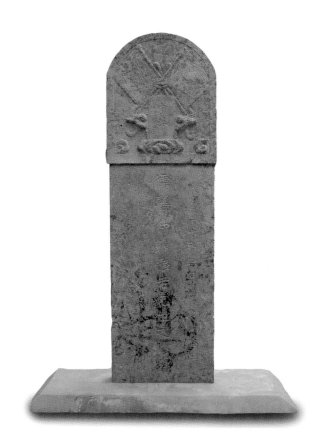

儒医仲镛强路碑

近代

石质

宽 65 厘米，厚 14.5 厘米，高 224.5 厘米

Road Tablet of Scholar-doctor Zhong Yongqiang

Modern Times

Stone

Width 65 cm/ Thickness 14.5 cm/ Height 224.5 cm

1938 年立石，碑身书"儒医仲镛强君路碑"

字样，为其后人所立。医药碑刻。完整无损。

陕西省宝鸡市征集。

陕西医史博物馆藏

The tablet, set up in 1938 by Zhong Yongqiang's descendants, is inscribed with Chinese characters meaning "Road Tablet of Revered Scholar-doctor Zhong Yongqiang". It was collected as a medical tablet in Baoji City, Shaanxi Province. It is still in good shape.

Preserved in Shaanxi Museum of Medical History

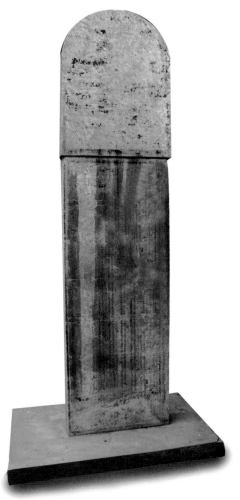

宝鸡海上方碑

近代

石质

宽 79 厘米，厚 23 厘米，高 310 厘米

Baoji Tablet of Hai Shang Fang Prescriptions

Modern Times

Stone

Width 79 cm/ Thickness 23 cm/ Height 310 cm

1946 年 12 月刻石并立碑。半圆形碑头。一碑四面，楷书，刻有"海上方"药方及当地民间验方 150 余首。医药碑刻。完整无损。陕西省宝鸡市虢镇磨性山征集。

陕西医史博物馆藏

The tablet, inscribed and set up in December 1946, has a semicircular top. On the four sides of the tablet are inscribed in regular script the selected prescriptions from the book "Hai Shang Fang" (*Hai Shang Fang Prescriptions*) and other 150 proved folk prescriptions. The item was collected as a tablet of medicine in Moxing Mountain, Guozhen Town, Baoji City, Shaanxi Province and is still in good shape.

Preserved in Shaanxi Museum of Medical History

集验良方碑

近现代

石质

宽 72 厘米，厚 25.5 厘米，高 310 厘米

Tablet of Collection of Valuable Proved Prescriptions

Modern times

Stone

Width 72 cm/ Thickness 25.5 cm/ Height 310 cm

1951 年立石。半圆形碑头。一碑四面，楷书当地名医验方及历代医家著作中部分名方 140 余首。医药碑刻。完整无损。陕西省宝鸡市虢镇景福山征集。

陕西医史博物馆藏

The tablet, set up in 1951, has a semicircular top. On the four sides of the tablet are inscribed in regular script a total of more than 140 proved prescriptions by the local famous doctors and from some of the works of doctors of the previous dynasties. It is in good shape. It was collected as a medical tablet in Fujing Mountain, Guozhen Town, Baoji City, Shaanxi Province.

Preserved in Shaanxi Museum of Medical History

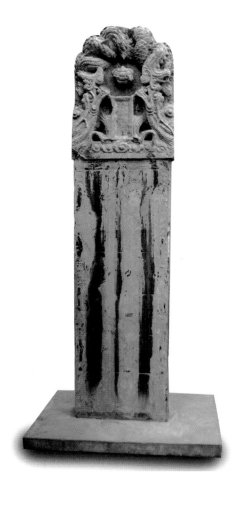

朱兴恭先生医方碑

近代

石碑

宽 76 厘米，厚 22.5 厘米，通高 312 厘米

Tablet of Dr. Zhu Xinggong's Prescriptions

Modern Times

Stone

Width 76 cm/ Thickness 22.5 cm/ Height 312 cm

碑头为二龙戏珠石雕，一碑四面刻石，楷书，
主要内容为近代骨伤科名医朱兴恭临证经验
方。完整无损。陕西省宝鸡市朱兴恭家人捐赠。

陕西医史博物馆藏

The head of the tablet is carved with two
dragons playing with a pearl. On the four sides
of the tablet are inscribed in regular script the
prescriptions of a celebrated modern doctor by
the name of Zhu Xinggong who specialized in
orthopedics and traumatology. It is still in good
shape. It was donated as a medical tablet by
Zhu Xinggong's family in Baoji City, Shaanxi
Province.

Preserved in Shaanxi Museum of Medical History

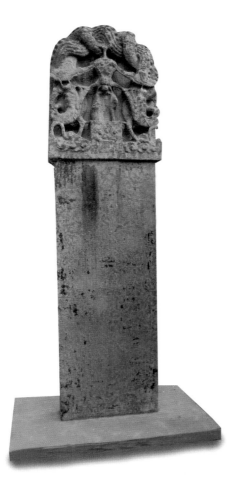

强和亭先生验方碑

近现代

石质

宽 79 厘米，厚 23 厘米，通高 303 厘米

Tablet of Dr. Qiang Heting's Prescriptions

Modern Times

Stone

Width 79 cm/ Thickness 23 cm/ Height 303 cm

碑头为龙寿石雕图，一碑二面，主要内容为
名医强和亭先生经验方。医药碑刻。完整无损。
陕西省宝鸡市强和亭家人捐赠。

陕西医史博物馆藏

The head of the tablet is carved with patterns
of dragon-like longevity. On the two sides of
the tablet are inscribed the prescriptions of a
celebrated modern doctor by the name of Qiang
Heting. It is still in good shape. It was donated
as a medical tablet by Qiang Heting's family in
Baoji City, Shaanxi Province,
Preserved in Shaanxi Museum of Medical History

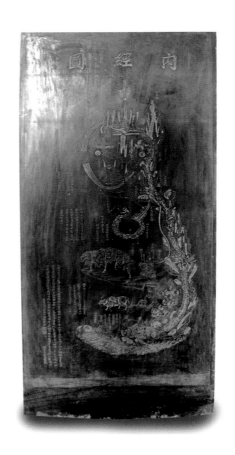

内经图

近现代

石质

宽 66 厘米，厚 9 厘米，高 150 厘米

Tablet of Neijing Diagram

Modern Times

Stone

Width 66 cm/ Thickness 9 cm/ Height 150 cm

原碑为清代，存于北京白云观。一碑两面，正面为《内经图》，另一面刻有孙思邈养生四言诗、扁鹊针病图及道教练功图说。完整无损。陕西医史博物馆复制。

陕西医史博物馆藏

The original tablet in the Qing Dynasty is in the White Cloud Taoist Temple in Beijing. Both sides of the tablet are inscribed. The front side is inscribed with *Neijing Diagram* while the back side is inscribed with Sun Simiao's four-line poems about health regimen, Bian Que's Acupuncture Diagram, and Illustration of Taoist Exercises. It is a replica made by Shaanxi Museum of Medical History, and is still in good shape.

Preserved in Shaanxi Museum of Medical History

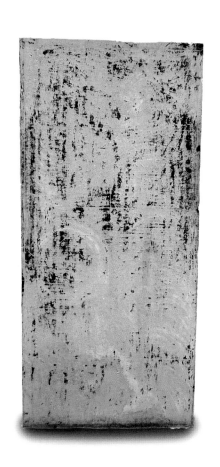

傅青主女科手迹

现代

石质

宽 63 厘米，厚 7 厘米，高 142.5 厘米

Tablet of Fu Qingzhu's Manuscripts on Female Diseases

Modern Times

Stone

Width 63 cm/ Thickness 7 cm/ Height 142.5 cm

碑为长方形，一碑两面，内容选录清代名医
傅山女科医方手迹。医药石刻。完整无损。
陕西医史博物馆刻碑。

陕西医史博物馆藏

On both sides of this rectangular tablet are
inscribed the selected original manuscripts on
female diseases by the famous doctor Fu Shan
in the Qing Dynasty. It is a tablet of medicine
carved by Shaanxi Museum of Medical History.
It is still in good shape.

Preserved in Shaanxi Museum of Medical History

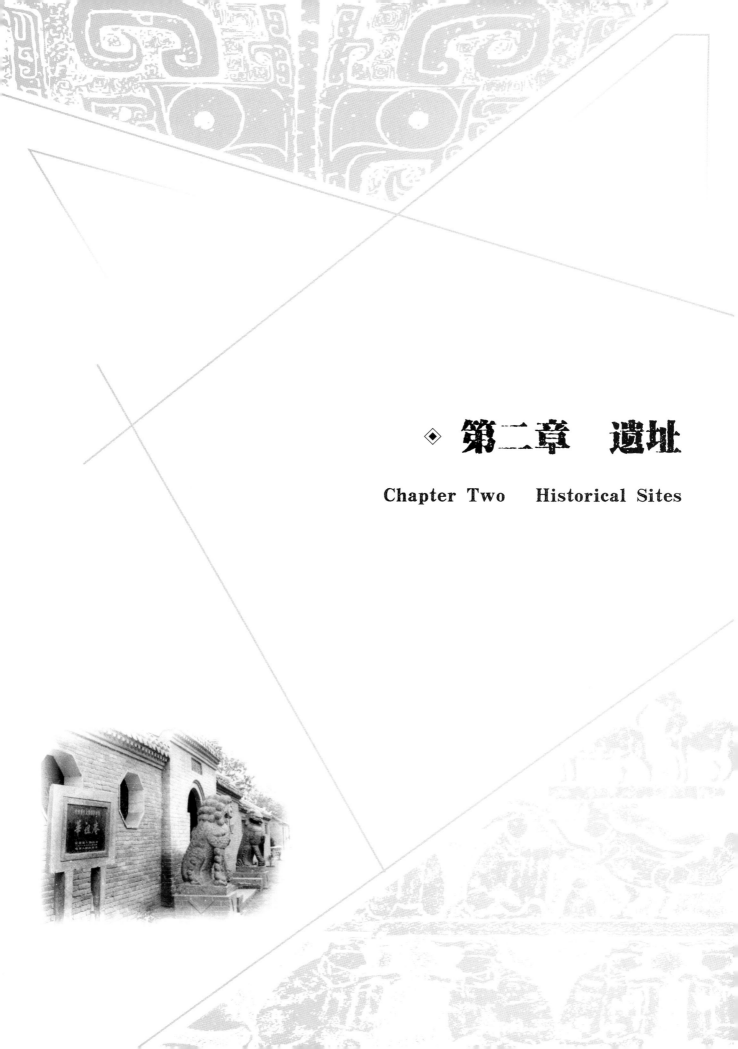

◇ 第二章　遗址

Chapter Two　Historical Sites

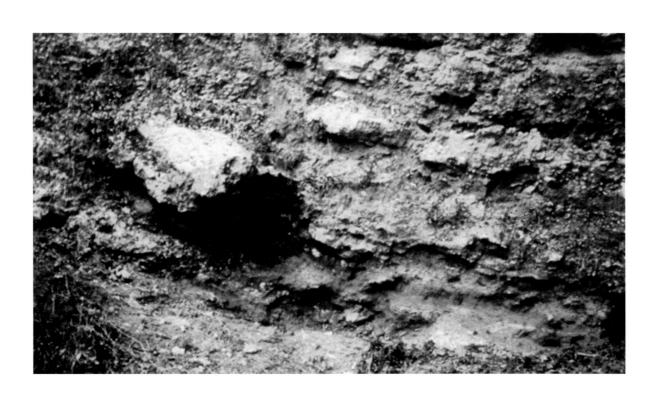

北京猿人居住遗址

该遗址 1927 年在北京市房山区周口店龙骨山发现，距今约 70 万—20 万年（旧石器时代）。北京猿人是中国代表性古人类之一。北京猿人已知用火和保存火种，而火的应用与人类健康有巨大关系。

Peking Man's Residence Site

The Peking Man's Residence Site was discovered on Longgu Mountain, Zhoukoudian, Fangshan District, Beijing in 1927. Peking Man inhabited this site approximately 700,000-200,000 years ago (The Paleolithic Age). Peking Man was one of the representatives of ancient humans in China. They knew the using and saving of fire, which had great impact on human health.

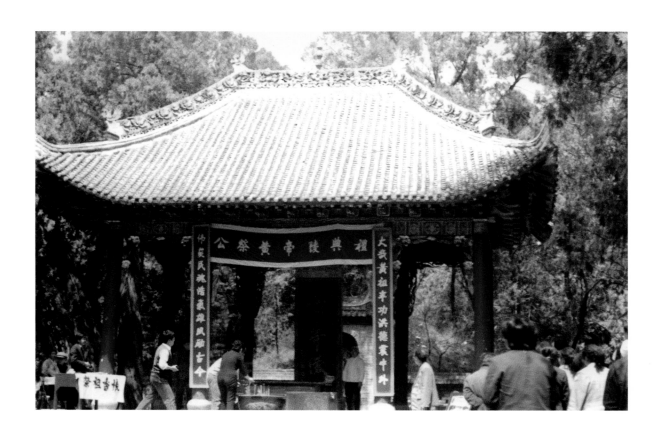

黄帝陵

黄帝陵位于陕西省黄陵县，是中华民族始祖黄帝轩辕氏的陵墓。1961 年，国务院公布为全国第一批重点文物保护单位。其号称"天下第一陵"，古称"桥陵"，为中国历代帝王和著名人士祭祀黄帝的场所。

Mausoleum of the Yellow Emperor

Located in Huangling County, Shaanxi Province, the Mausoleum, also known as "Qiao Mausoleum", is for Xuan Yuan the Yellow Emperor, a legendary ancestor of the Chinese nation. In 1961, it was enrolled as the national key cultural relic (the first batch). Famed as "the first mausoleum in the world", it has witnessed sacrificial ceremonies held by the emperors and celebrities through all the dynasties.

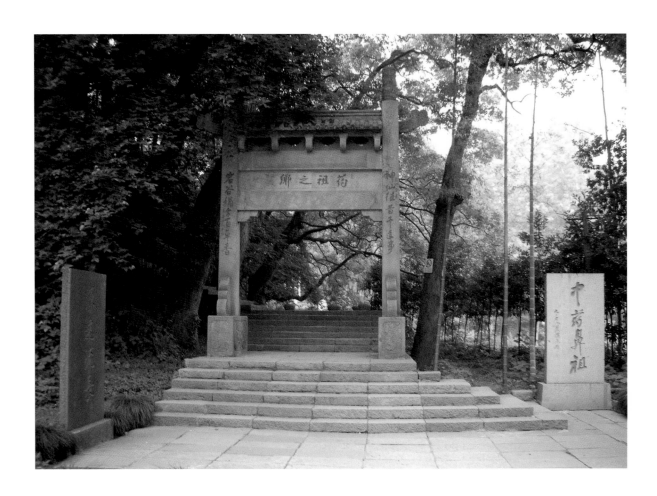

桐君山

药祖圣地桐君山位于浙江省桐庐县富春江畔。桐君为黄帝时人。黄帝命桐君与巫彭采药求道，至桐庐县东山侧隈桐树下居住，旁人问其姓名，指树下茅庐回答，时人呼其为桐君，此山与县因而得名。

朱德明提供

Tong Jun Mountain

Tong Jun Mountain, a sacred residence of medicine forefathers, is situated by Fuchun River in Tonglu County, Zhejiang Province. The folktale goes that Tong Jun, a legendary figure in the Yellow Emperor's time, gathered herbs and pursued Taoism with Wizard Peng at the Yellow Emperor's service. When in Tonglu, he dwelt under a phoenix tree (which is pronounced as "tong" in Chinese). Some neighbors asked him for his name, and were responded with a silent allusion to the tree. Then he was honorably addressed as "Tong Jun" (a noble man of phoenix trees), from which the mountain nearby and the county were named after.

Provided by Zhu Deming

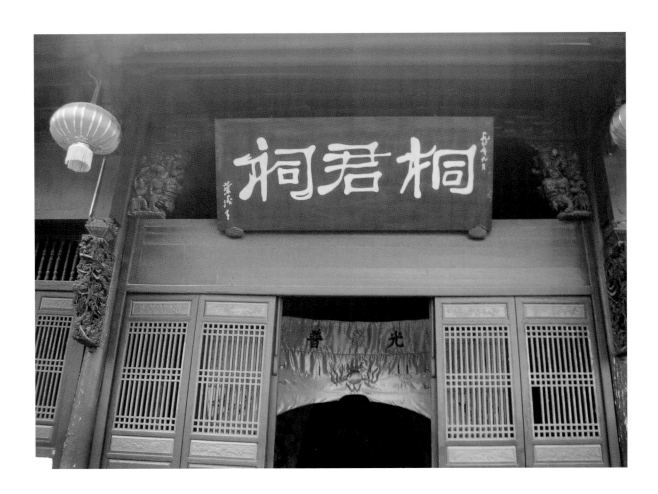

桐君祠遗址

桐君祠位于浙江省桐庐县富春江畔药祖圣地桐君山。黄帝命桐君与巫彭采药求道，至桐庐县东山侧隈桐树下居住，旁人问其姓名，指树下茅庐回答，时人呼其为桐君，此山与县因而得名。

朱德明提供

Tong Jun Temple Site

The Temple is situated at Tong Jun Mountain, a sacred residence of medicine forefathers, by Fuchun River in Tonglu County, Zhejiang Province. The folktale goes that Tong Jun, a legendary figure in the Yellow Emperor's time, gathered herbs and pursued Daoism with Wizard Peng at the Yellow Emperor's service. When in Tonglu, he dwelt under a phoenix tree (which is pronounced as "tong" in Chinese). Some neighbors asked him for his name, and were responded with a silent allusion to the tree. Then he was honorably addressed as "Tong Jun" (a noble man of phoenix trees), from which the mountain nearby and the county were named after.

Provided by Zhu Deming

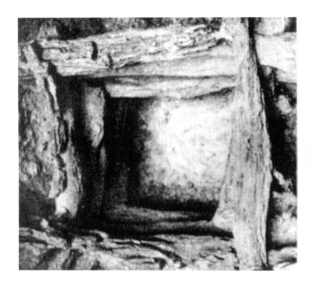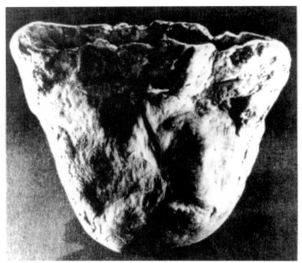

水井遗址、汲水桶

商

木质

汲水桶：口径 24.8 厘米，高 23.7 厘米

Well Site, Dip-bucket

Shang Dynasty

Wood

Dip-bucket: Mouth Diameter 24.8 cm/ Height 23.7 cm

汲水桶现于井底，扁椭圆口，状似盔形，系用一块木瘿子掏成。两侧有对称的圆孔，用以系绳汲水。水井遗址共二眼，位于房基附近。1973 年发现于河北藁城台西村商代遗址。

When unearthed, the helmet-shaped dip-bucket was found to be on the bottom of the well. With a flat oval mouth, it was hollowed out from a tree root. There were two symmetrical round holes on both sides for the convenience of fastening ropes to fetch water from the bottom of the well. In 1973, two well sites were discovered near the foundation of a house on Shang Site in Taixi Village, Gaocheng District, Hebei Province.

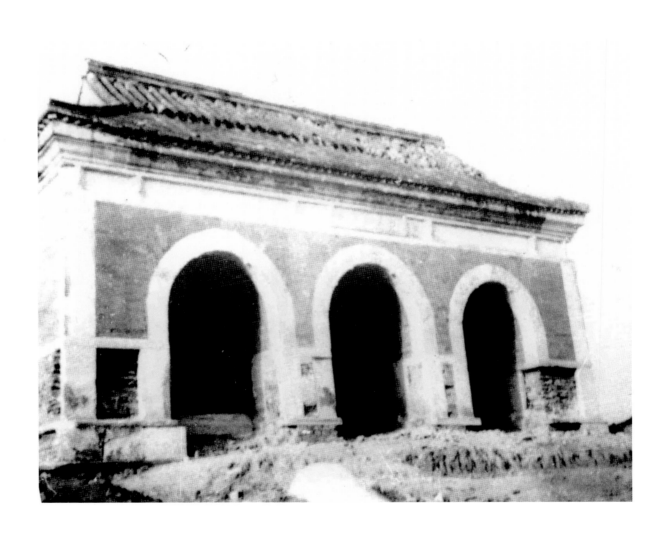

河北任丘药王庙外景

纪念战国时期名医扁鹊的陵庙有多处，其中较为著名的是河北任丘药王庙。后历经沧桑，仅存白石砌成的三座山门，门额分别刻有"敕建药王庙"、"敕建三皇殿"、"敕建文昌阁"等字样。此为 1954 年所摄。

中国医史博物馆供稿

Exterior Scene of Temple of King of Medicine

There are too many temples enshrining and worshiping Bian Que, the famous doctor in the Warring States Period, among which the temple in Renqiu of Hebei Province is well-known. After surviving many vicissitudes, only three gates made of white stones of this temple still remain. On the lintels of the gates were respectively engraved words meaning "Temple of King of Medicine Built with the Imperial Decree", "Three-emperor Hall Built with the Imperial Decree" and "Wenchang Pavilion Built with the Imperial Decree". This photo was taken in 1954.

Provided by China Museum of Medicine

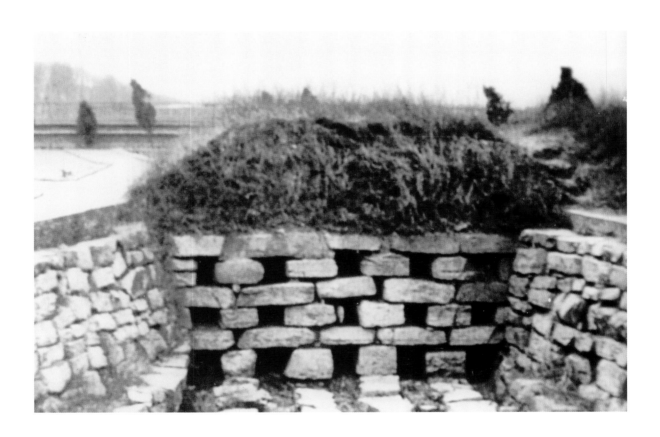

临淄齐故城下水道

战国时期

临淄齐故城内的排水明渠，在通往城外穿过城墙时用石块砌成外宽内窄的涵洞。此图摄自大城西部一条水渠的出口。

山东博物馆供稿

Sewer of Former Qi Capital of Linzi

Warring States Period

The photo shows an open sewer channel for drainage in Linzi, the former capital of Qi Kingdom. The channel was transformed into a culvert made of stones with wide exterior and narrow interior when it was to go through the city wall. The picture was taken from the exit of a water channel in the west of the former capital.

Provided by Shandong Museum

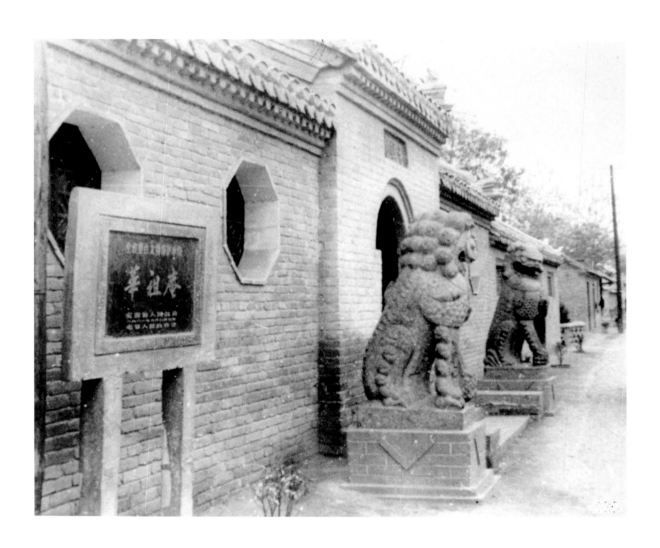

华祖庵

图为华佗故里——安徽亳州之华祖庵门景。华祖庵是祭祀我国东汉时期杰出的医药学家华佗的庙祠。华佗字元化，名敷，安徽亳州人，精通岐黄。其创用"麻沸散"施行外科手术，为外科鼻祖。其创编"五禽戏"，开创我国体育医疗的先河。

Hua Tuo's Hut

The picture shows the gate of Hua Tuo's Hut in Bozhou, Anhui Province. It is an ancestral temple to offer sacrifices to Hua Tuo, an outstanding physician in the Eastern Han Dynasty, whose style name is "Yuanhua" and given name "Fu". He was born in Bozhou, Anhui Province, and he was proficient in Chinese herbal medicines. Initially applying "Ma Fei San" (anesthesia powder) to operations, he was honored as "the Forefather of Surgery". And he was the first advocator of exercise therapy by originating "the Five-animal Boxing".

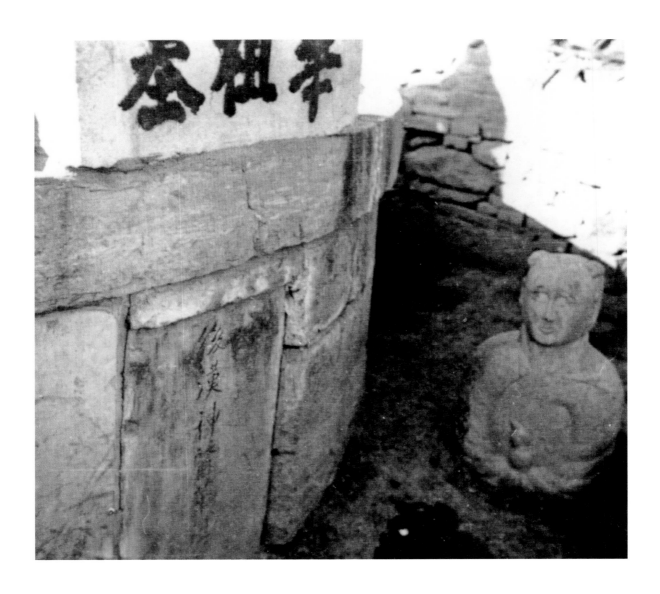

徐州华佗墓

该墓位于江苏徐州彭城路华祖庙侧，是华佗的衣冠冢。华佗（约145—208），字元化，沛国谯（今安徽亳州）人。东汉名医，首创手术麻醉药"麻沸散"。

Hua Tuo's Tomb in Xuzhou

The tomb is next to Hua Tuo's Temple at Pengcheng Road, Xuzhou, Jiangsu Province. Actually it is his cenotaph. Hua Tuo (about 145–208), with "Yuanhua" as his style name, was born in Qiao of the Pei Kingdom (an ancient city, now known as Bozhou in Anhui). He was a prestigious physician in Eastern Han Dynasty, well known as the initiator of "Ma Fei San" (anesthesia powder).

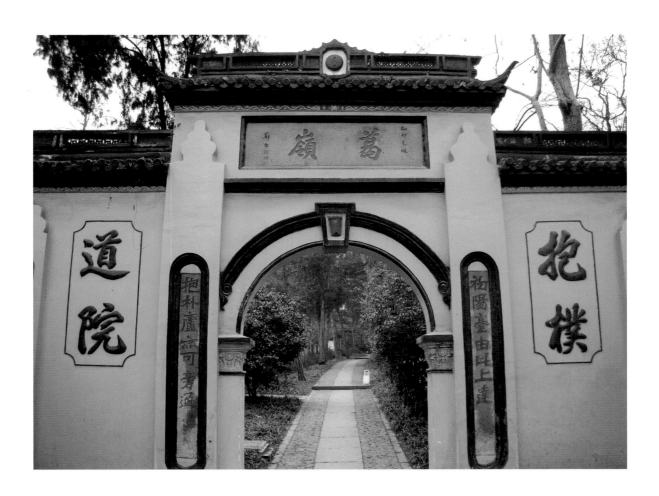

葛岭

杭州北山葛岭，因葛洪炼丹而得名，今洗药池、
炼丹井等古迹尚存。

朱德明提供

Mount Geling

Mount Geling, located at Beishan Mountain
in Hangzhou, has been famous for Ge Hong's
alchemy. Nowadays, there are still some historic
sites, such as the Medicine Washing Pool and
the Alchemy Well.

Provided by Zhu Deming

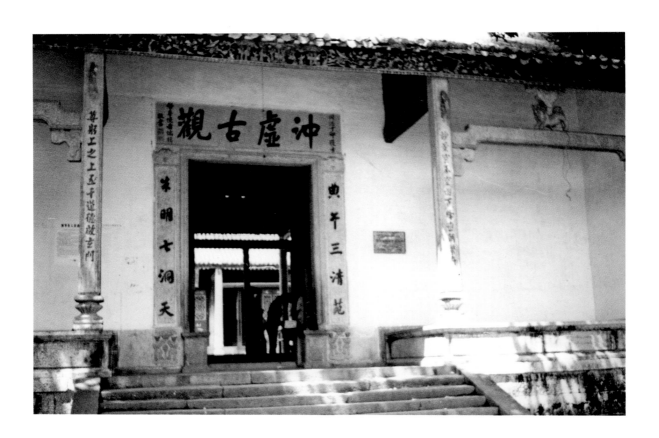

冲虚观门景

冲虚观位于今广东省罗浮山。相传葛洪在此道观炼丹。原址为东晋名医葛洪所建四庵之一的南庵，初名都虚，后改为冲虚。唐置祠，宋立观。观后有稚川丹灶遗址、洗药池、朱明洞等名胜古迹。

Gate of Chongxu Taoist Temple

It is said that Ge Hong, a well-known alchemist in Eastern Jin Dynasty, made pills of immortality in this Taoist temple which is located in Luofu Mountain, Guangdong Province. Primitively, at the site Ge Hong built South Hut, one of his four huts. Then it was named as "Duxu", and finally as "Chongxu". It was converted into an ancestral hall in Tang Dynasty, and established as a Taoist temple in Song Dynasty. Behind the Temple are relics such as Zhichuan's (Ge Hong's style name) Alchemical Furnace, Medicine Pond, and Zhuming Grotto.

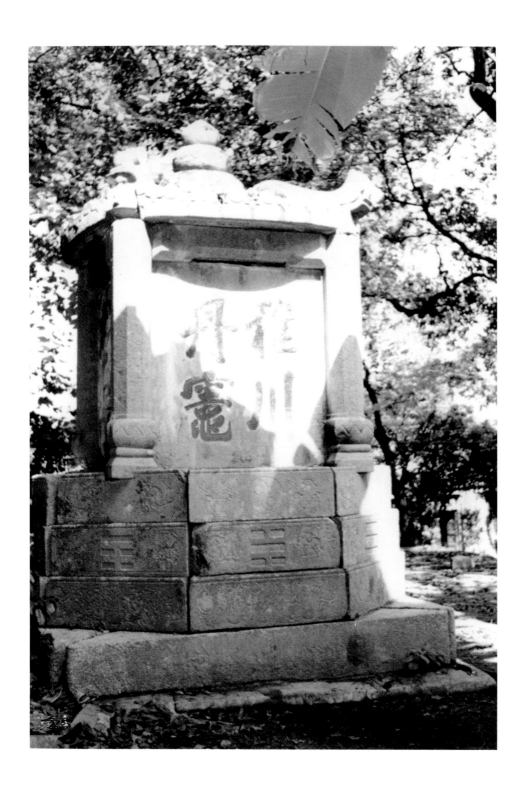

稚川丹灶

花岗岩质

基座直径 1.5 米，高 2 米

此丹灶传为葛洪炼丹用灶。"稚川丹灶"4
字据考系东坡书法。

Alchemy Furnace with Characters "Zhi Chuan Dan Zao"

Granite

Pedestal Diameter 1.5 m/ Height 2 m

It is said that the furnace was the very alchemy furnace used by Doctor and Alchemist Ge Hong of the Eastern Jin Dynasty because it has the characters "Zhi Chuan Dan Zao", which are identified through investigation as Su Dongpo's handwriting.

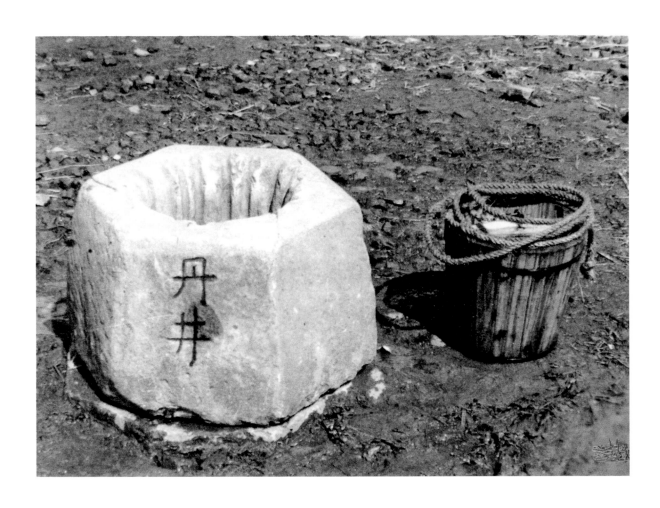

葛洪炼丹用井

直径 0.48 米，高 6.4 米

此井位于江苏句容城隍庙内，据当地人相传为
葛洪炼丹用井，建于东晋。诗人李白曾为该井
作诗记载。井上有井圈，呈六角形，上刻"丹井"、
"灵雨仙泉"、"道光乙未"等字样。

Ge Hong's Alchemical Well

Diameter 0.48 m/ Height 6.4 m

The well is sited in the Temple of City God,
Jurong, Jiangsu Province. Sunk in Eastern Jin
Dynasty, it was said to have been used by Ge
Hong in his alchemy. Li Bai, a prestigious poet
in the Tang Dynasty, depicted the well in one of
his poem. The well is curbed by a hexagon ring.
On the ring is engraved characters such as "Dan
Jin" (Alchemical Well), "Lin Yu Xian Quan"
(Immortal's Spring), and "Dao Guang Yi Wei" (the
year of 1825, in the reign of Emperor Daoguang).

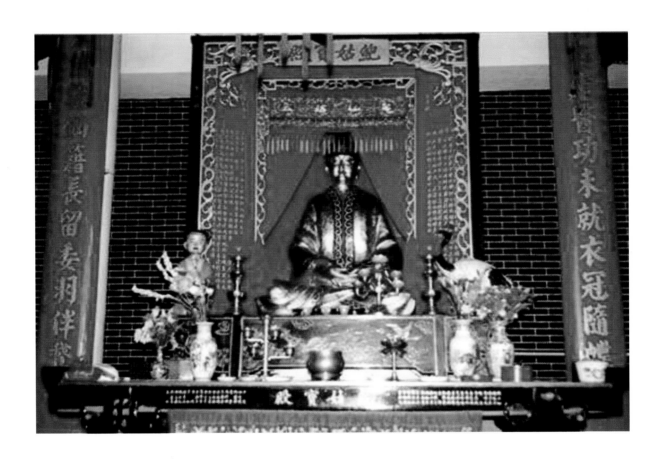

鲍姑宝殿

鲍姑为葛洪妻，是我国最早的女灸家。南海越秀山有鲍姑井，又名"虬龙古井"；有赘艾，即红脚艾，鲍姑用井泉水与红脚艾为医方活人无数。鲍姑相传升仙后，三元宫设祠供奉。

Bao Gu's Shrine

Bao Gu, wife of Doctor and Alchemist Ge Hong of the Eastern Jin Dynasty, is the female pioneer of moxibustion in China. Bao Gu Well, also called "Ancient Qiu Long Dragon Well", is in Yuexiu Mountain in the former South China Sea area. Bao Gu had saved innumerable lives of people by using this wellspring and the Chinese mugwort. After becoming immortal, Bao Gu was enshrined and worshiped in the Sanyuan Taoist Temple.

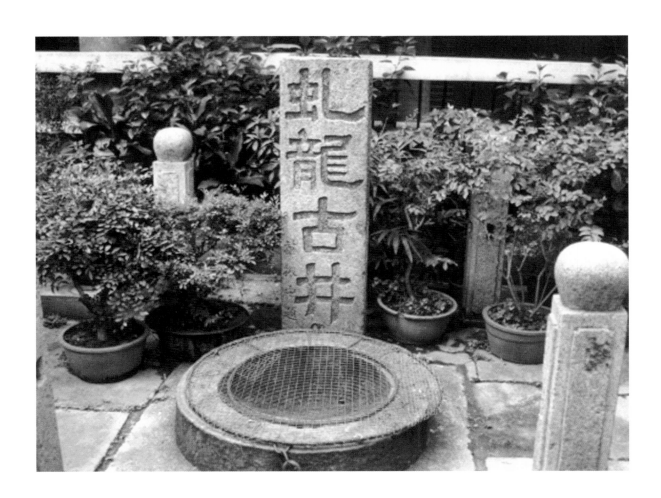

虬龙古井（鲍姑井）

鲍姑为葛洪妻，是我国最早的女灸家。南海越秀山有鲍姑井，又名"虬龙古井"；有赘艾，即红脚艾，鲍姑用井泉水与红脚艾为医方活人无数。鲍姑相传升仙后，三元宫设祠供奉。

Ancient Qiu Long Dragon Well (Bao Gu Well)

Bao Gu, wife of Doctor and Alchemist Ge Hong of the Eastern Jin Dynasty, is the female pioneer of moxibustion in China. Bao Gu Well, also called "Ancient Qiu Long Dragon Well", is in Yuexiu Mountain in the former South China Sea area. Bao Gu had saved innumerable lives of people by using this wellspring and the Chinese mugwort. After becoming immortal, Bao Gu was enshrined and worshiped in the Sanyuan Taoist Temple.

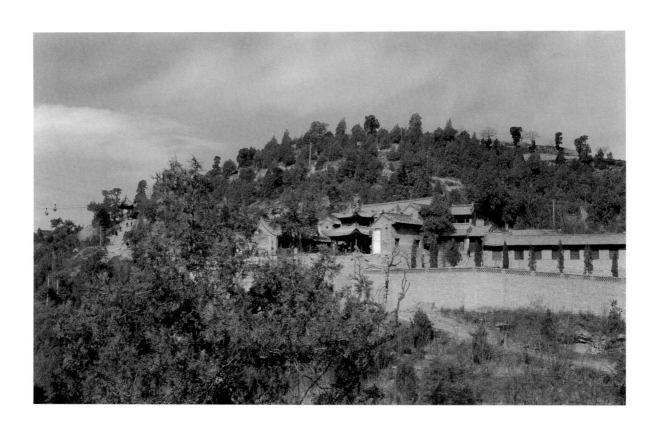

陕西耀州区药王山外景

药王山位于陕西省铜川市耀州区，是唐代著名医学家孙思邈长期隐居的地方，因民间尊奉孙思邈为"药王"而得名。孙思邈，陕西耀州区孙家塬人，编著《千金要方》《千金翼方》各30卷，对中国医药学发展做出了杰出的贡献。

King of Medicine's Mountain in Yaozhou District, Shaanxi Province

In Yaozhou District, Tongchuan City, Shaanxi Province, the Mountain was inhabited by Sun Simiao—an outstanding pharmacist in Tang Dynasty—in his seclusion, thereby it was named after him for his reputation as the "King of Medicine". Sun Simiao, born in Yaozhou District, Shaanxi Province, had compiled *A Thousand Invaluable Prescriptions* and *Supplement to a Thousand Invaluable Prescriptions* (30 volumes each). He had contributed remarkably to traditional Chinese medicine.

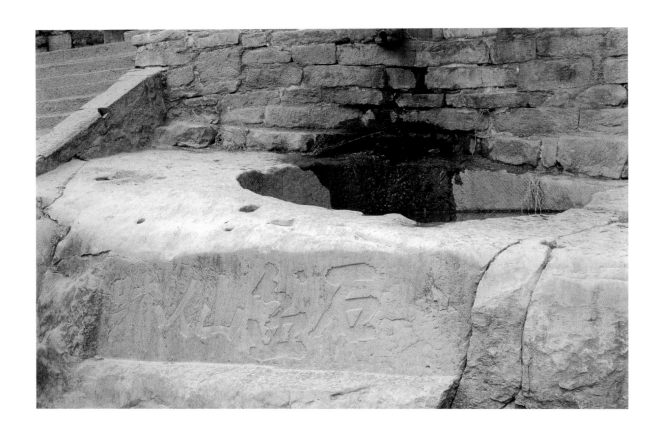

洗药池

该池相传为孙真人洗药之池，又名洗药盆。逢雨池满。柏子、柏叶浸其中，水绿沉甘洌，夏不秽，冬不涸。池外题字"石盆仙迹"，为明代进士邑人左经书。洗药池位于陕西省耀州区药王山。

Herb Washing Pond

It is said that Sun Simiao used to wash herbs in the pond, which is also called a basin. When it rains, the pond will be full. If cedar seeds and leaves are soaked in the water, it turns green, limpid, sweet and refreshing. The merit of the pond is that it will not become dirty in summer and not get dry in winter. The outside of the pond is inscribed with "Shi Pen Xian Ji" meaning "stone basin used by True Man Sun" written by a local scholar with the surname of Zuo, a successful candidate in the highest imperial examinations in the Ming Dynasty. The pond is situated in King of Medicine's Mountain, Yaozhou District, Shaanxi Province.

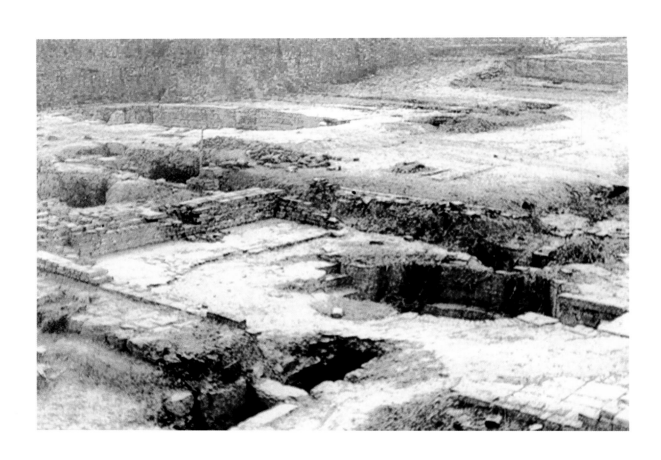

华清宫遗址

宫内有5个石浴池，即文献所记星辰汤、贵妃汤、太子汤、莲花汤和尚食汤。图为1982—1985年发掘的浴池遗址原貌。该遗址位于陕西临潼骊山北麓。

Huaqing Palace Site

There are five stone pools in this palace, which, as documents have recorded, are Xingchen Pool, Guifei Pool, Taizi Pool, Lianhua Pool and Shangshi Pool. The picture above shows the original appearance of the pools being excavated between 1982 and 1985. The site is located at the northern foot of Lishan Hill in Lintong District, Shaanxi Province.

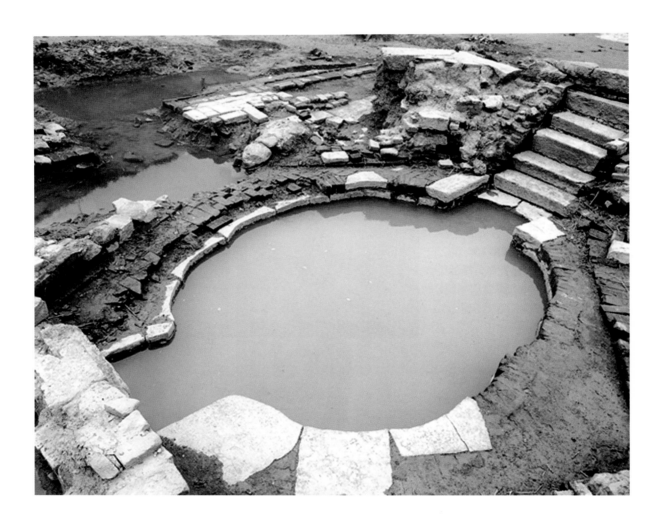

贵妃池

该遗址系唐玄宗李隆基赐给杨贵妃沐浴的汤池，因形似一朵盛开的海棠花而又名海棠汤。图为 20 世纪 80 年代初发现的贵妃池遗址原貌。该遗址位于陕西省西安市临潼区华清池。

Guifei Pool

Guifei Pool (Imperial Concubine's Pool) is also named as Haitang Pool because its shape looks like a blooming Chinese flowering crabapple, whose pronunciation in Chinese is "haitang". It was granted by Emperor Xuanzong Li Longji of the Tang Dynasty for his concubine Yang Guifei to bathe. The picture above shows the original appearance of the Guifei Pool site when it was discovered in the early 1980s. The site is located in Huaqing Pool, Lintong District, Xi'an City, Shaanxi Province.

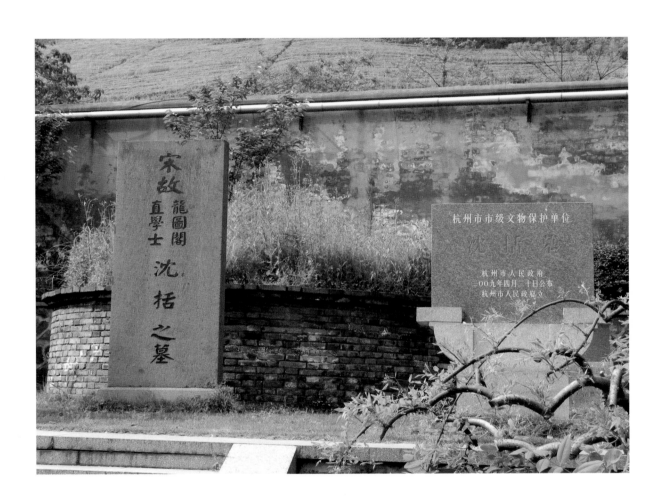

沈括墓

北宋著名的医药学家杭州人沈括 (1031—
1095) 墓，地处杭州市余杭区安溪太平山
下。

朱德明提供

Shen Kuo's Tomb

Shen Kuo was the distinguished
pharmacologist in Northern Song Dynasty.
He was buried at his hometown, at the foot
of today's Taiping Mountain, Anxi Village,
Yuhang District of Hangzhou.
Provided by Zhu Deming

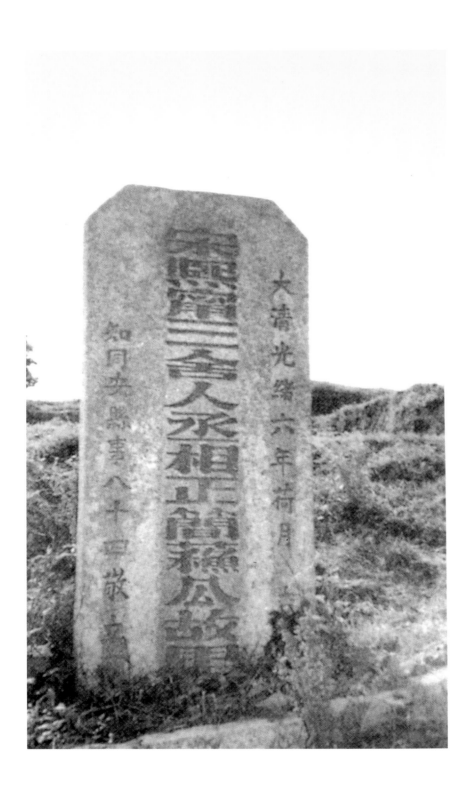

苏颂故里碑

苏颂（1020—1101），北宋官吏兼天文学家、药学家。苏颂字子容，原籍泉州南安（今属福建），后徙居丹阳（今江苏南京），曾参与校注《嘉祐补注神农本草》，又主编《本草图经》。此碑为光绪六年（1880）所立。

Monument of Su Song's Hometown

Su Song(1020–1101), also named Zi Rong, was not only an official but also an astronomer and pharmaceutical scientist in the Northern Song Dynasty. His ancestral home was in Nan'an, Quanzhou (now in Fujian Province), but later he moved his family to Danyang (now in Nanjing, Jiangsu Province). He once participated in checking and annotating Jia You Bu Zhu Shen Nong Ben Cao(An Added Annotation to Shennong Materia Medica Done in Jiayou Period) and was editor-in-chief of "Ben Cao Tu Jing" (Illustration of Materia Medica). This monument was set up in the sixth year of Guangxu's Reign of the Qing Dynasty(1880).

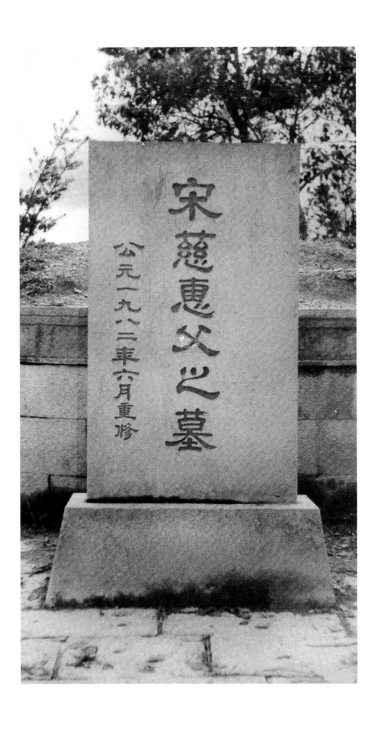

宋慈墓地

宋慈（1186—1249），宋代法医学家，字惠父，福建建阳人。其数十年深谙法医检验之道，又博采诸书。

Song Ci's Tomb

Song Ci (1186-1249), also named Hui Fu, was a famous forensic scientist in Song Dynasty in Jianyang, Fujian Province. He was well read and well versed in forensic examination.

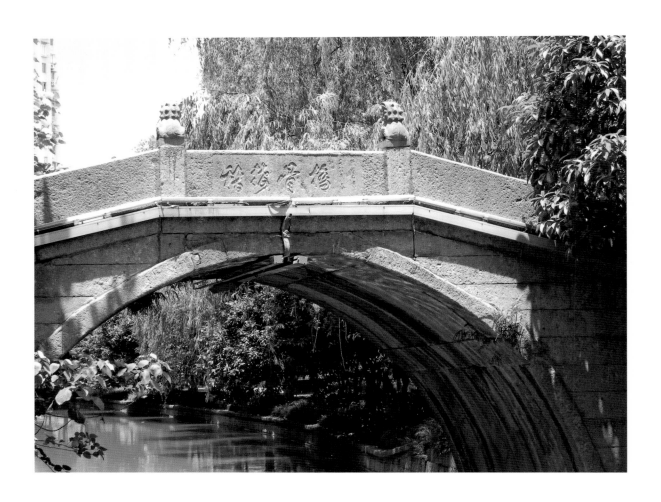

嵇接骨桥

嵇清是南宋杭州一位"善疗金疮骨损"的骨科名医。民间相传他的药铺开在中河东面，门口没有桥相通。在政府的资助下，人们在药铺门口的中河上造一座桥，以便患者就医。人们把这座桥称为"嵇接骨桥"。

朱德明提供

Dr. Osteosynthesis Ji Bridge

Ji Qing was a famous doctor who was good at osteosynthesis in Hangzhou in Southern Song Dynasty. It was said that there was no bridge in front of his herbal medicine shop which was at the eastern bank of the river, so the government granted to build a bridge to offer the patients convenience. And the bridge was called Dr. Osteosynthesis Ji Bridge.

Provided by Zhu Deming

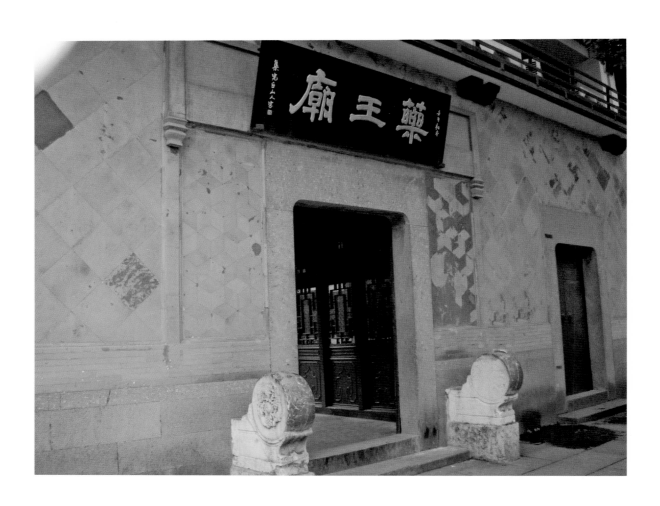

吴山药王庙遗址

位于浙江省杭州市吴山的药王庙，建于南宋初年。清康熙十八年 (1679) 国药业商定在吴山药王庙每年神农氏诞生日（农历九月初九）集会一次，借以联系业务。

朱德明提供

Site of King of Medicine's Temple Temple at Wushan Mountain

The temple, built in the early years of Southern Song Dynasty, stands at Wushan Mountain, Hangzhou, Zhejiang Province. In the 18th year under the reign of Emperor Kangxi of Qing Dynasty (1679), the TCM trades picked the temple to hold their annual business session on the 9th day of the 9th month of the Chinese lunar year, the birthday of the first ancestor of herbal medicine Shennong.

Provided by Zhu Deming

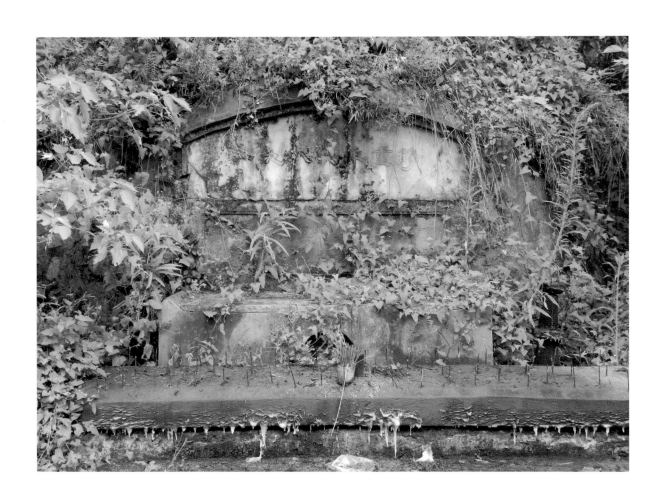

楼英墓

楼英（1320—1389），浙江萧山人。楼英曾拜朱丹溪为师。洪武中，游金陵，曾为朱元璋诊病，"具合上意"。欲官以太医院，以老病故辞，获重赏而归，隐于仙岩洞。他积 30 多年功力，编成《医学纲目》39 卷巨著等。

朱德明提供

Tomb of Lou Ying

Lou Ying (1320-1389) was born in Xiaoshan, Zhejiang Province. He learnt from Zhu Danxi. When he was travelling in Jinling in the Hongwu period of Ming Dynasty, he cured Emperor Zhu Yuanzhang successfully and the emperor was quite satisfied. The emperor wanted to entitle him as an officer in the royal hospital, but Lou Ying persistently refused the offer by giving an excuse of his old age. In the end, he was permitted to go back to Xianyan Cave with a large amount of money and awards. With his 30 years experience, he wrote a 39-volume "Yi Xue Gang Mu" (*Compendium of Medicine*).

Provided by Zhu Deming

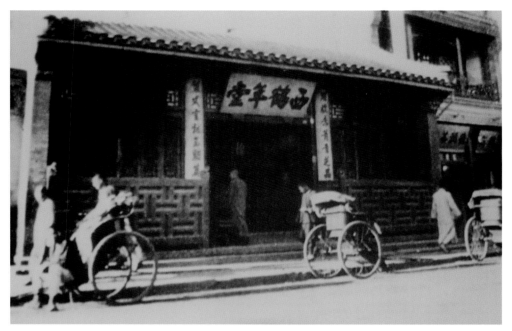

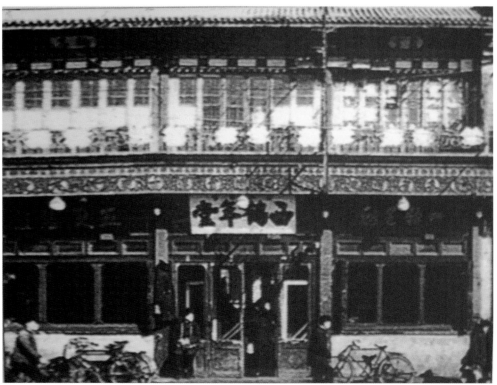

北京鹤年堂

北京鹤年堂始建于明永乐三年 (1405)，位于北京市宣武区（现西城区）菜市口大街铁门胡同迤西路北，骡马市大街西口，与丞相胡同相对，与回民聚居的牛街相邻。中华人民共和国成立后，1954 年公私合营，鹤年堂被并于宣武区医药公司，"文革"后鹤年堂又恢复老字号品牌。本图摄于 2017 年 4 月。

刘学春提供

Beijing He Nian Tang Pharmacy

The pharmacy, founded in the third year during the reign of Emperor Yongle of Ming Dynasty(1405), stands at the north of Yixi Road, Tiemen Lane, Caishikou Street of Xuanwu District, Beijing. West to Luomashi Street and opposite to Chengxiang Lane, the store is adjacent to Niu Street, a Mohammedan neighborhood. In 1954 after the founding of the People's Republic of China, the store was merged as a joint venture with the state by Xuanwu Pharmaceutical Co. The store regained its time-honored brand after the ending of the Cultural Revolution in 1976. The picture was taken in April 2017.

Provided by Liu Xuechun

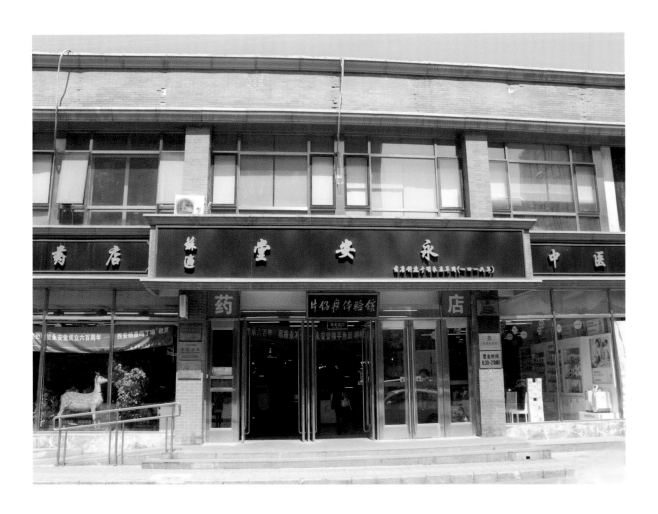

北京永安堂

永安堂药店始建于明朝永乐年间 (1403—
1424)，位于北京东四牌楼东西角（现北京市
东城区朝内大街366号）、1956年公私合营。
"文革"期间，改名为"曙光药店"。1988年，
恢复原称。1993年秋，在原址上改建重修。
本图摄于2017年4月。

刘学春提供

Beijing Yong An Tang Pharmacy

Yong An Tang Pharmacy, founded during the
reign of Emperor Yongle of the Ming Dynasty
(1403–1424), stands at Dongsi Pailou in Beijing
(No. 366, Chaonei Street, Dongcheng District).
It was nationalized and jointly run by the state
and the private section since 1956 and renamed
as "Shuguang Drugstore" in the Cultural
Revolution. It regained its time-honored brand
in 1988, and was restored at the old site in the
autumn 1993. The picture was taken in April
2017.

Provided by Liu Xuechun

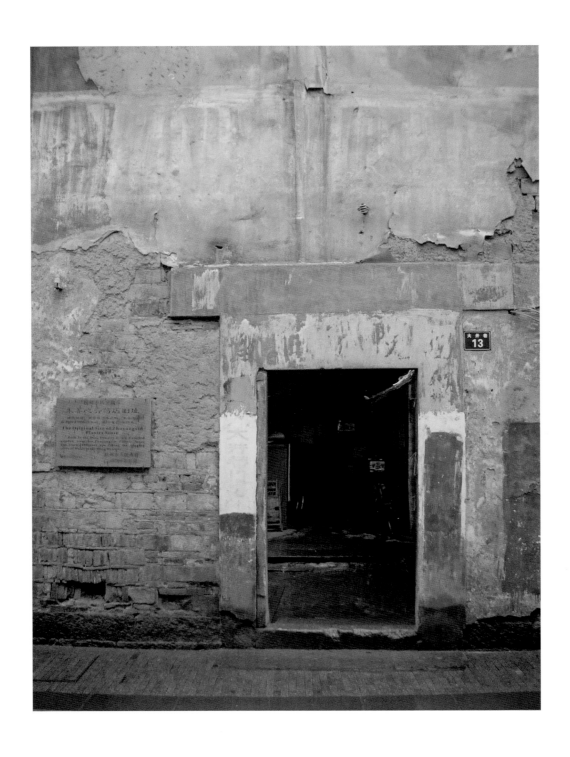

朱养心药室西门

明万历年间（1573—1620），伤外科医家朱养心，从余姚迁居杭州，在浙江省杭州市大井巷口开设朱养心丹膏店，为5开间店面，东、西两个墙门出入。

朱德明提供

West Gate of Zhu Yangxin's Pharmacy

Zhu Yangxin, a trauma surgeon, moved from Yuyao to Hangzhou in Wanli period (1573–1620) of Ming Dynasty. He used to run Zhu Yangxin Pharmacy, which consisted of five linked rooms with one door on the eastern wall and the other on the western wall going around Dajing Alley, Hangzhou, Zhejiang Province.
Provided by Zhu Deming

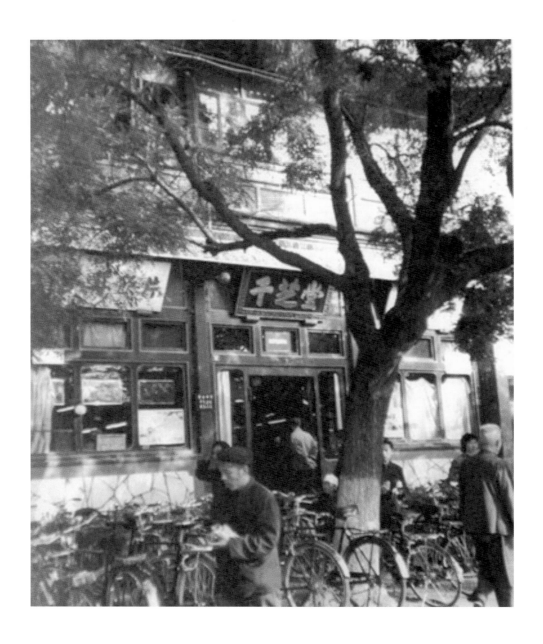

北京千芝堂旧址

北京千芝堂开业于明朝万历年间（1573—1620），旧址位于崇外大街 48 号，现金伦大厦所在地。据《南城医药业》所述，千芝堂在最初的几百年里一直生意平平，到了 19 世纪下半叶已无法继续营业。清光绪七年 (1881)，专营药材批发的吴霭亭用 2000 两白银买得千芝堂铺底。原建筑为一座传统的三间门面开间两层小楼，前店后厂，雕梁画栋，金碧辉煌，楼前牌匾上的"千芝堂"三字为吴霭亭亲笔书写。著名古建专家郑孝燮曾赞叹，千芝堂的建筑格局与梁上精致的彩画对研究明清古代建筑有很大的参考价值。

刘学春提供

Site of Beijing Qian Zhi Tang Pharmacy

Qian Zhi Tang Pharmacy started the business during the reign of Emperor Wanli of the Ming Dynasty (1573–1620). As documented in *Nancheng Medicine*, the business kept jogging along over hundreds of years, and was on the verge of bankruptcy in the late 19th Century. In 1881 (the seventh year during the reign of Guangxu Emperor of Qing Dynasty), Wu Aiting, a drug wholesale merchant, bought off the store for 2000 taels of silver and became its new owner. The old two-story house was traditionally three-bayed, the front as the store and the backyard as the workshop. It was splendidly and magnificently decorated with carved beams and painted pillars. The overhead plaque was inscribed with three Chinese characters "Qian Zhi Tang" written by Wu himself. Zheng Xiaoxie, a prestigious expert at historic buildings once admirably remarked that the layout and exquisite beam paintings were especially valuable for researches into old-style buildings in Ming and Qing Dynasties.

Provided by Liu Xuechun

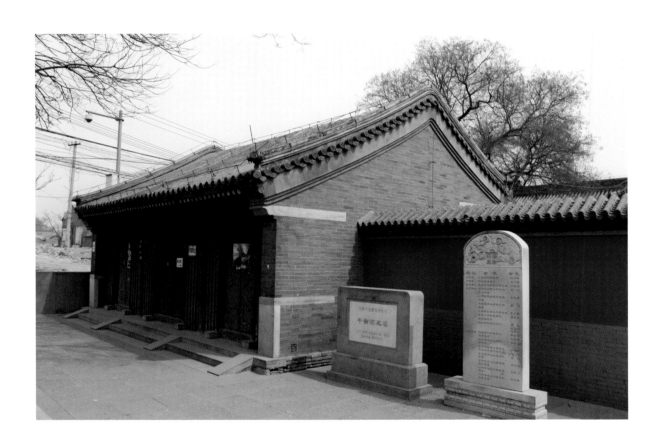

丰台药王庙

丰台药王庙始建于明代，清乾隆三十三年 (1768) 重修，现位于北京市丰台区花乡（看丹桥十字路口向西 1 公里处）。该庙坐西朝东，西南门处有直径近 2 米的明代古槐 1 棵，庙内有药王殿、三皇殿、娘娘殿等建筑，以及两座碑刻。在药王殿山墙两处镶嵌着《重修药王庙碑文》和京城各界香客修庙捐款名单。现存庙宇保存完整。本图摄于 2017 年 4 月。

刘学春提供

Fengtai Temple of King of Medicine

Built in the Ming Dynasty, the temple was restored in the 33rd year under the reign of Emperor Kangxi of the Qing Dynasty. In Huaxiang, Fengtai District of Beijing (1 km away west to the crossroad of Kandan Bridge), the temple faces south, with an old Chinese scholar-tree of 2 m in diameter outside the south-west gate. In the temple are Halls of King of Medicine, Three Emperors, and Empresses, as well as two stone tablets. On the gables of the Hall of King of are Medicine inscribed *An Memorandum on Restoring the Temple* and a list of the donating pilgrims. The temple is now fully preserved. The picture was taken in April 2017.

Provided by Liu Xuechun

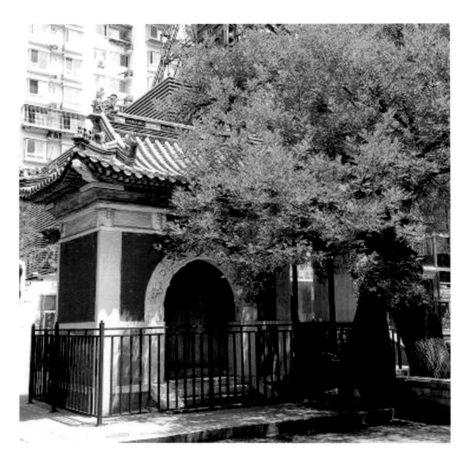

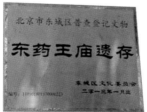

东药王庙遗存

北京东直门药王庙遗存俗称"东药王庙",明万历四十五年(1617),位于东直门内大街与东直门北中街南口相交的丁字路口东北侧(北京市东城区东直门北中街南口路东,东直门内大街 5 号)。2002 年,该处出土残碑一块。碑身长 2.4 米,宽 1.07 米,厚 0.5 米,螭首,额篆"敕建东药王庙碑铭"。楷书碑数百字,记载了明万历年间修建东药王庙的史实,落款"大明万历岁在丁巳孟秋吉日立"。

刘学春提供

Relics of Eastern Temple of King of Medicine

Known as "Eastern Temple of King of Medicine" in the folk, the temple was built in the 45th year under the reign of Emperor Wanli of the Ming Dynasty. The temple stands at the north-east side of the cross of Dongzhimen Nei Street and Dongzhimen Bei Street (S.) (at No. 5 of Dongzhimen Nei Street). In 2002, a tablet residue (2.4 m in length, 1.07 m in width, and 0.5 m in thickness) was unearthed, atop with a legendary dragon chi's head on which is carved in seal character *An Inscription of Imperial Edict for Building the Eastern Temple of Medicine King*. The front of the tablet was inscribed in regular script of several hundred words about the history of the building of the temple in Wanli period, ending with characters saying that "it was founded on the lucky day in the third month of the Autumn of 1617 of Wanli Period." The construction is fully recorded on the tablet.

Provided by Liu Xuechun

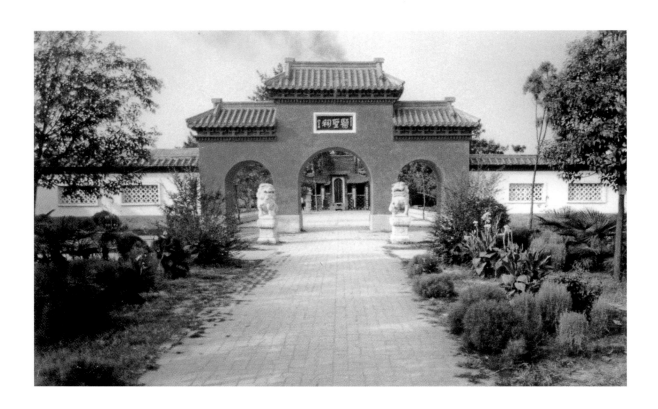

南阳医圣祠外景

清顺治十三年（1656），为纪念医圣张仲景，于河南南阳城东张仲景墓故址修建医圣祠，并重修墓地，立碑记事。其后，又经多次扩建。医圣祠有正、偏两院，正院墓门前有圣祖庙、故里碑亭，后为仲景墓；偏院有内经楼、医圣井等 20 多座建筑。图为 1981 年整修后的医圣祠外景，远处为仲景墓及碑。

Exterior Scene of Temple of Sage of Medicine

In the thirteenth year of Shunzhi's Reign of the Qing Dynasty (1656), Temple of Sage of Medicine was constructed on former site of Zhang Zhongjing's tomb to the east of Nanyang City, Henan Province. Later the tomb was reconstructed and a monument was set up to keep a record of all the related events. Thereafter, the temple has been expanded several times and finally built into two yards. In the main yard, the Temple of Sage of Medicine and the Stele Pavilion stand in front of the gate, while Zhang Zhongjing's tomb lies behind the gate. In the side yard, there are more than 20 buildings including the Library Pavilion, and Well of the Sage of the Medicine. This picture shows the exterior scene of the Temple of Sage of Medicine after its renovation in 1981, with Zhang Zhongjing's tomb and monument in the distance.

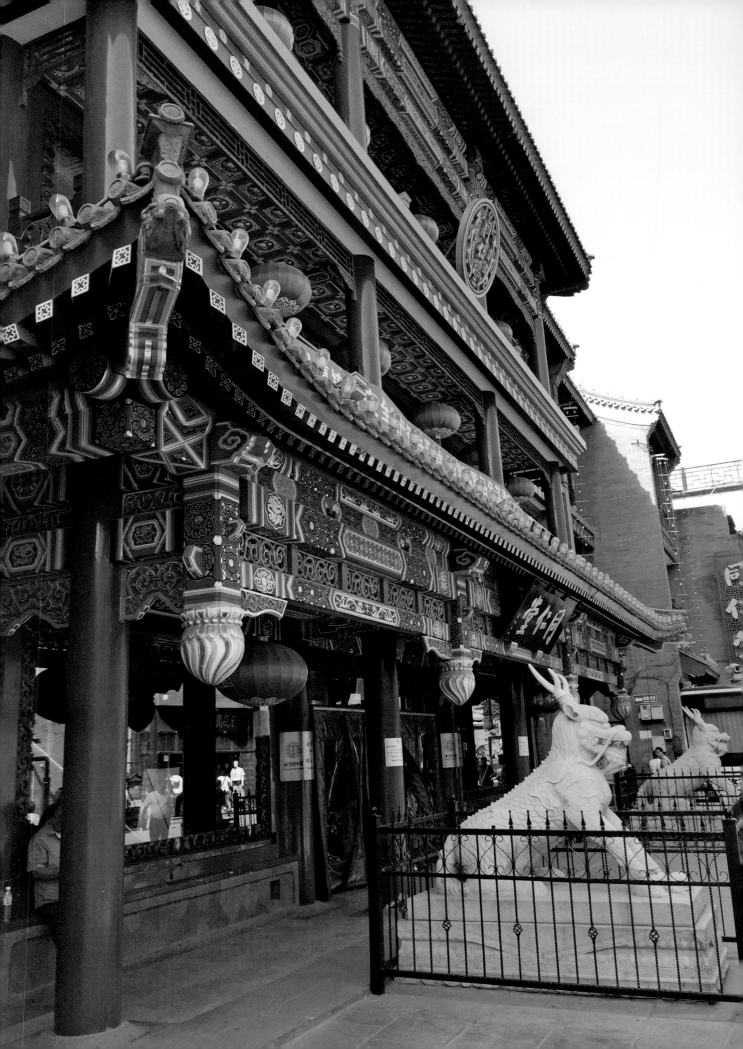

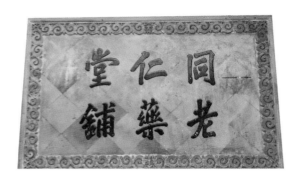

北京同仁堂

北京同仁堂创建于清康熙八年（1669），位于北京市前门大栅栏路南。雍正元年（1723）被钦定供奉清宫御药房用药，独办官药。恪守"炮制虽繁必不敢省人工，品味虽贵必不敢省物力"的传统古训，以"配方独特、选料上乘、工艺精湛、疗效显著"而享誉海内外。2006 年，同仁堂中医药文化被列入国家非物质文化遗产名录。本图摄于 2014 年 8 月。

刘学春提供

Beijing Tong Ren Tang Pharmacy

Tong Ren Tang Pharmacy was founded in the 8th year under the reign of Emperor Kangxi of the Qing Dynasty (1669) at the southern end of the present day Dashilaner Road in Beijing. In 1723 it was imperially appointed as an official supplier of the royal pharmacy. Strictly adhering to the doctrine that "drugs must be fully and carefully processed with no mercy for labors and costs", it is reputable at home and abroad for its "curative druggery uniquely formulated and finely processed from qualified materials". In 2006, the pharmacy was enlisted as National Intangible Cultural Heritage. The picture was taken in August 2014.

Provided by Liu Xuechun

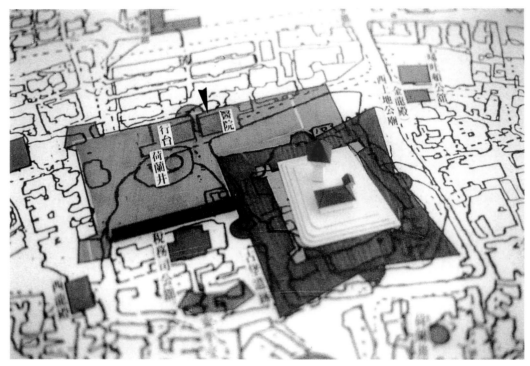

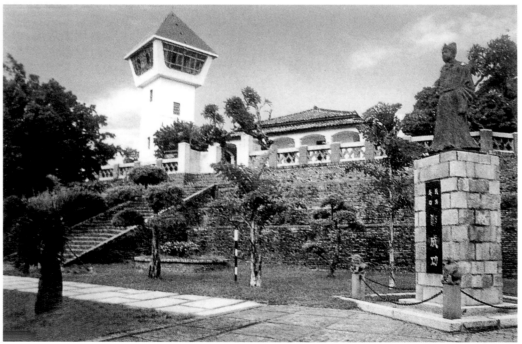

台湾地区明代之医院示意图

荷兰于 1624 年入侵台湾地区，在台南登陆，占领安平，随即在安平开设商馆，上图为安平古堡陈列室内之热兰遮城（安平）模型。外城（长方形部分）临海，为贸易区，外城设有医院。图中箭头所示为医院旧址之方位。下图为安平古堡今貌，右边铜像为郑成功。

哈鸿潜供稿

Diagram of Hospital in Taiwan in the Ming Dynasty

Holland landed in Tainan and trespassed Taiwan of China in 1624, and then occupied Anping where they soon established trade offices. The upper picture shows the model of Zeelandia (Anping) City. The outer city (the rectangular section), close to the sea, was the trade zone where a hospital was set up. The arrow in the picture points to the former site of the hospital. And the lower picture is of today's Anping Castle, to the right of which is the bronze statue of Zheng Chenggong.

Provided by Ha Hongqian

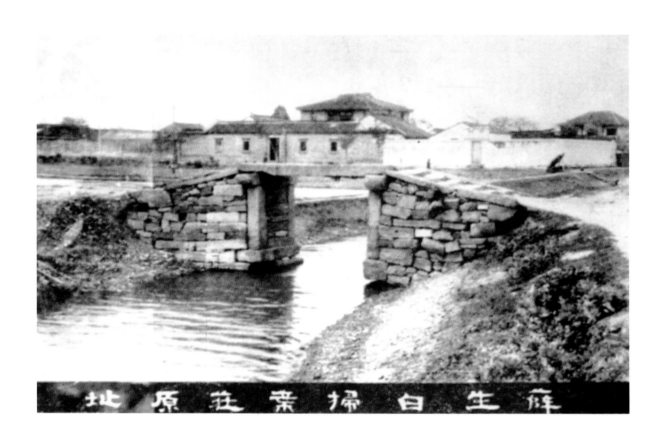

薛雪扫叶庄原址

薛雪（1681—1770），字生白，号一瓢，又号槐云道人、磨剑道人、扫叶山人，江苏吴县（今苏州市）人。薛雪善诗工画，尤精于医，著有《湿热病篇》等。图为薛氏所居扫叶庄原址（今苏州医学院所在地）。

Xue Xue's Former Residence "Saoye Zhuang"

Xue Xue(1681–1770), also named Sheng Bai, who styled himself Yi Piao or Taoist Huaiyun, or Taoist Mojian, or Recluse Saoye, was from Wu County (now as Suzhou City), Jiangsu Province. He was good at poems and painting, especially well-known for his medical practice. He wrote many medical books, including "Shi Re Bing Pian" (*On Diseases Caused by Damp and Heat*). The picture shows Xue Xue's former residence Saoye Zhuang. (Suzhou Medical College stands here today.)

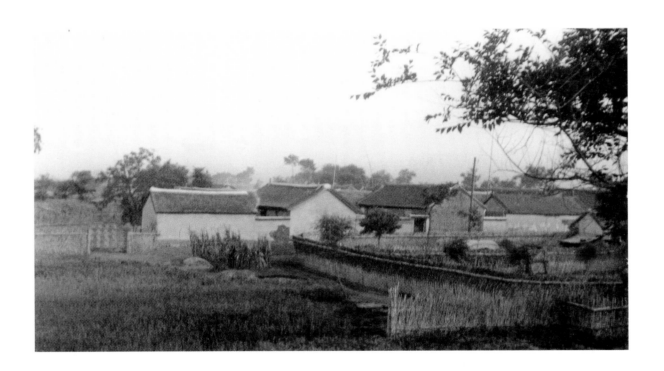

王清任故里

其位于河北省玉田县雅鸿桥河东村。王清任（1768—1831），又名全任，字勋臣，我国清代的解剖学家、医学家，著有《医林改错》，在我国医学史上占有重要地位。图为王清任故里鸦鸿桥镇之一角。

Wang Qingren's Hometown

Wang Qingren (1768–1831), with an alternative given name as Quanren and a style name as Xunchen, was an anatomist and physician in the Qing Dynasty. Also the author of "Yi Lin Gai Cuo" (*Correction on Errors in Medical Classics*), he is influential in Chinese medical history. The picture shows his hometown East Yahongqiao Village, Yutian County, Hebei Province.

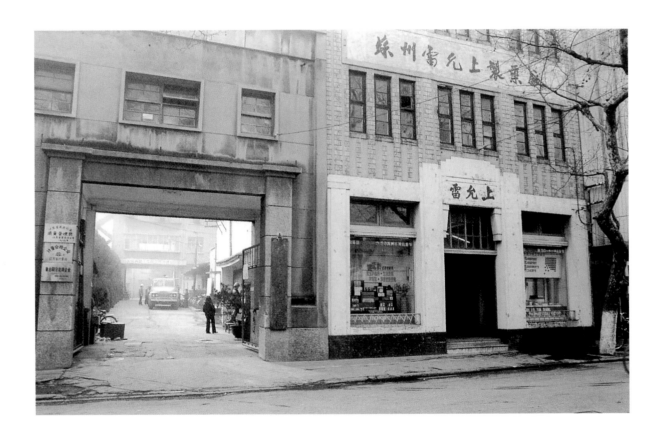

苏州雷允上药店

该药店为雷允上创立,坐落于苏州老阊门内闹市区,以制售六神丸、行军散、痧药、蟾酥丸、玉枢丹、辟瘟丹等细料成药而蜚声海内外,是一家具有250余年历史的著名药铺。雷氏于乾隆初行医、制药于"诵芬堂",集医药于一处。人们合并其医名与铺名,故有"雷允上诵芬堂"之称。

Lei Yunshang's Pharmacy in Suzhou

The pharmacy, located in the downtown of Laochangmen in Suzhou, was initiated by Lei Yunshang. It was a famous herbal medicine shop with a history of more than 250 years, and was renowned both at home and abroad mainly for the manufacturing and selling of such fine patent medicines as Liushen Miraculous Pills, Xingjun Medicinal Powder, Cholera Medicine, Dry Toad Venom Pill, Yushudan Pellet, and Plague Pellet, etc. He practiced medicine at the beginning of Qianlong's Reign of the Qing Dynasty and made medicine in "Song Fen Tang". Combining his name and the name of his pharmacy, people call it "Lei Yunshang's Song Fen Tang".

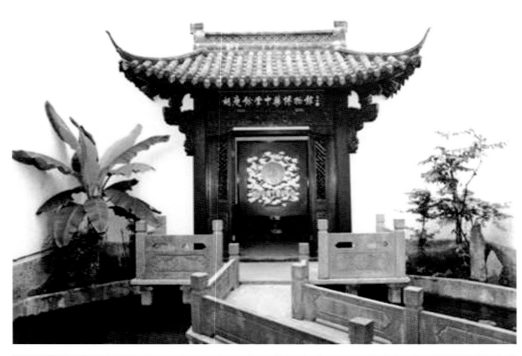

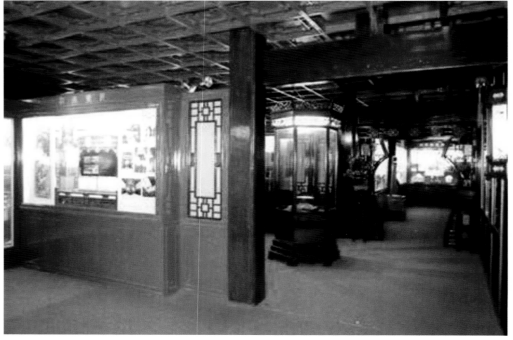

杭州胡庆余堂中药博物馆

胡庆余堂中药博物馆位于浙江省杭州市大井巷。同治十三年（1874），清末著名红顶商人胡雪岩创立胡庆余堂，被誉为"江南药王"。1987年，胡庆余堂在古建筑内创办了中药博物馆。上图为门景，下图为内景。

Hu Qing Yu Tang Traditional Chinese Pharmacy Museum in Hangzhou

The museum sits at Dajin Lane, Hangzhou, Zhejiang Province. In the 13th year of the reign of Emperor Tongzhi in Qing Dynasty (1874), Hu Xueyan, a distinguished merchant official of higher ranks, founded Hu Qing Yu Pharmacy, for which he was reputed as "Medicine King in Jiangnan "(area south to the Yangtze River). The Pharmacy Museum was established in some of the old buildings of Hu Qing Yu Tang in 1987. The top picture shows the entrance and the bottom shows the inner.

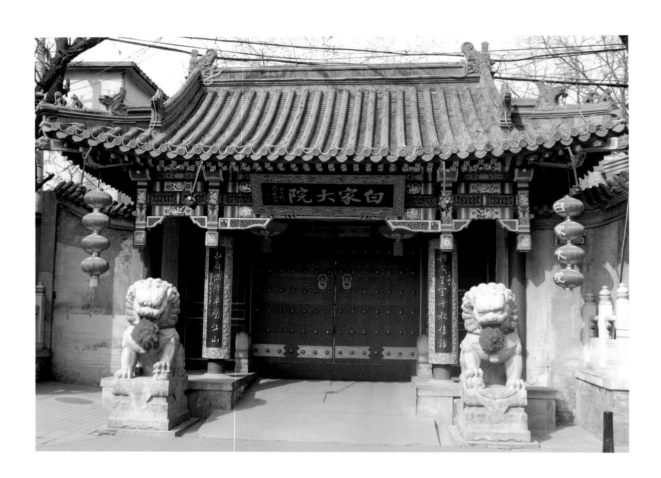

北京同仁堂分号宏德堂旧址

北京同仁堂分号宏德堂旧址位于北京海淀区苏州街29号，原是第四代礼亲王杰书于康熙年间建造的"礼亲王花园"。民国初年，转给了同样声势赫赫的同仁堂乐家的乐静宜，更名为"乐家花园"，开设北京同仁堂分号宏德堂。中华人民共和国成立后，该院由北京八一中学使用。现原址为白家大院餐厅。本图摄于2017年4月。

刘学春提供

Site of Hong De Tang As a Branch of Beijing Tong Ren Tang Pharmacy

Located at No. 29, Suzhou Street, Haidian District, Beijing, Hong De Tang once was Prince Li Qin's Garden built by Prince Li Ⅳ (Jie Shu) in years under the reign of Emperor Kangxi of the Qing Dynasty. In the early time of Republic of China, it was taken over by Le Jingyi, a celebrity from the Le's — master boss of Tongrentang. Renamed as "Le's Garden", it was then reestablished as a branch of Tongrentang in the name of "Hong De Tang". After the founding of the People's Republic of China, the yard was converted into a campus of Bayi Middle School. At present, a restaurant, Ba's Courtyard, runs at the former site. The picture was taken in April 2017.

Provided by Liu Xuechun

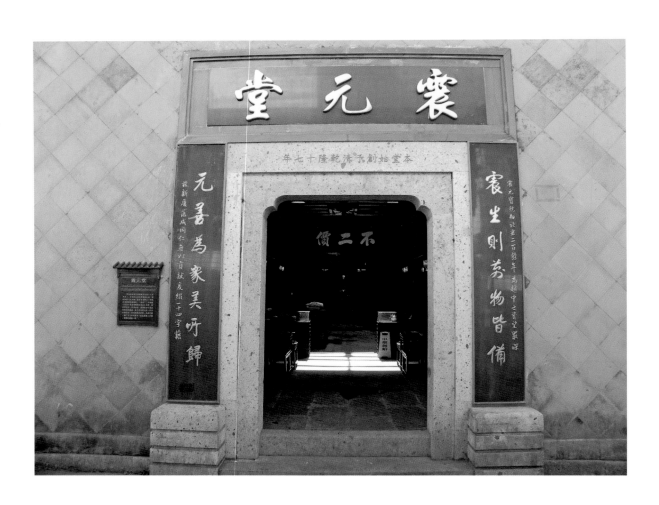

震元堂遗址

震元堂药店创始于清乾隆十七年（1752），
由杜景湘开设在浙江省绍兴市城内水澄桥下。
中华人民共和国成立前，外柜门市，内柜拆
兑，前店后场，经营中药饮片、丸散、人参、
鹿茸、燕窝、银耳等 1200 个品种。

朱德明提供

Site of Zhen Yuan Tang Pharmacy

Zhen Yuan Tang Pharmacy was started by Du
Jingxiang in the 17th year (1752) under the
reign of Emperor Qianlong of the Qing Dynasty.
It stood by Shuicheng Bridge in Shaoxing City.
Before the founding of the People's Republic
of China, it dealt with as many as 1,200
products as herbal pieces, pills, powders, and
restoratives. The front houses provided services,
whereas the backyard processed medicines.
Provided by Zhu Deming

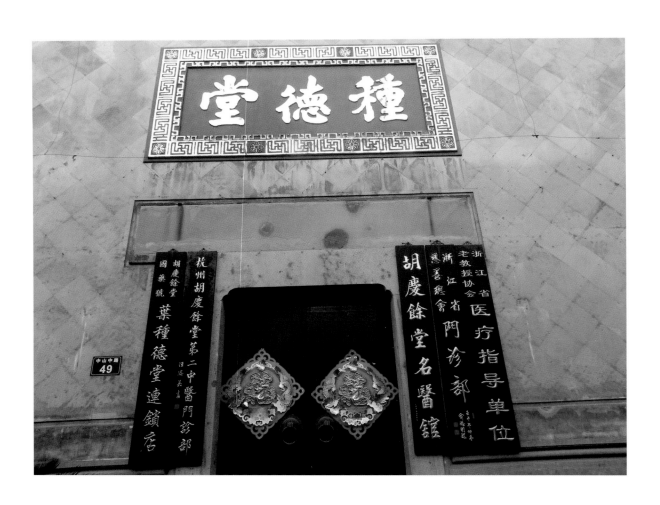

叶种德堂

杭州叶种德堂国药号创始于清嘉庆十三年
(1808)，是一家开设较早、规模较大，自制
丸散膏丹，经营各地地道药材，声誉远达浙、
赣、皖、闽各省的国药号。

朱德明提供

Ye Zhongde Tang Pharmacy

Hangzhou Ye Zhongde Tang Pharmacy was
initiated in the 13th year (1808) under the
reign of Emperor Jiaqing of the Qing Dynasty.
It specialized in homemade medicines (pills,
pellets, plaster, and powder) and crude drugs.
As one of the earliest and biggest pharmacies,
it enjoyed good reputations in the eastern
provinces of Zhejiang, Jiangxi, Anhui and
Fujian of China.

Provided by Zhu Deming

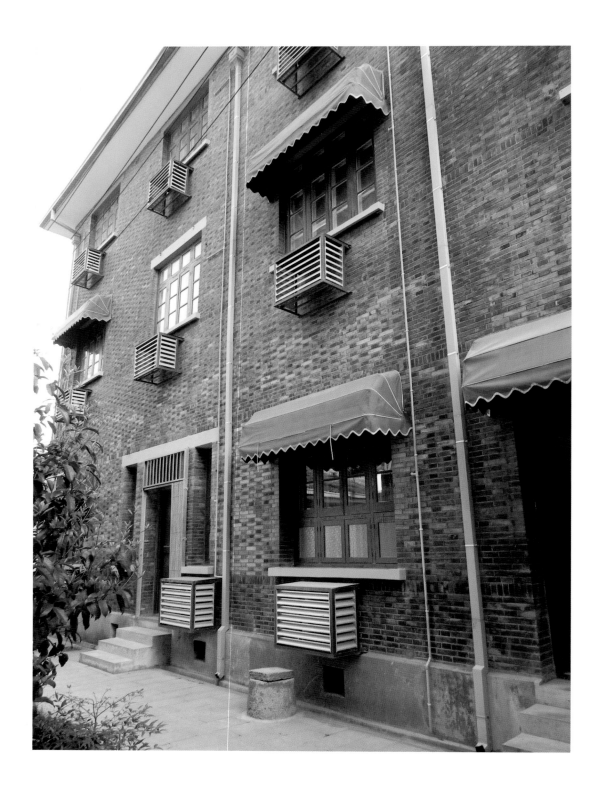

仁爱医院天主教堂遗址

1868 年，天主教仁爱会修女在天汉洲桥（今中山北路）创立仁爱会医院分院，称"仁慈堂"。民国十七年（1928）1 月 6 日，法籍天主教修女郝格助在刀茅巷 222 号创办杭州仁爱医院，今杭州市红十字会医院。

朱德明提供

Site of Charity Hospital Cathedral

In 1868, Catholic nuns of the Missionaries of Charity founded "Ren Ci Tang", a branch of Charity Hospital at Tianhanzhou Bridge (now the North Zhongshan Road). And Sr. Hacard, a French Catholic nun, founded Hangzhou Charity Hospital, now the Hangzhou Red Cross Hospital, at No. 222 Daomao Alley on January 6, 1928.

Provided by Zhu Deming

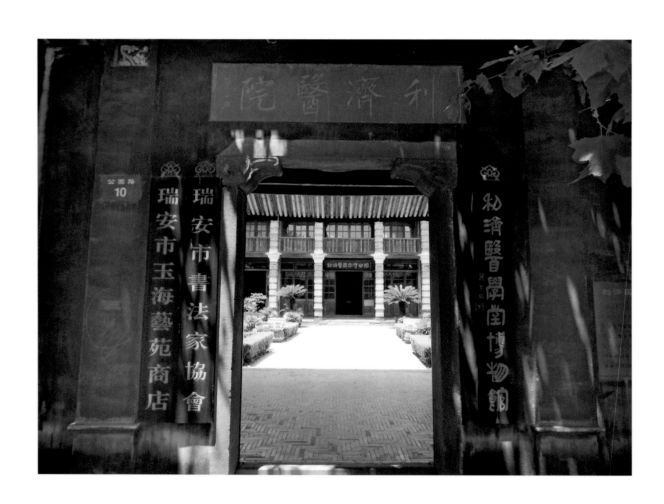

利济医院遗址

清光绪十一年（1885），陈虬等创办瑞安利济医院，院址在浙江省瑞安杨衙里，为温州首所具有相当规模和较高水平的中医医院。

朱德明提供

Site of Liji Hospital

Chen Qiu founded Liji Hospital in Ruian with others in 1885, the eleventh year under the reign of Guangxu of the Qing Dynasty. Located at Yangyali, Ruian, Zhejiang Province, it was the first hospital of traditional Chinese medicine with considerable scale and relatively high level in Wenzhou.

Provided by Zhu Deming

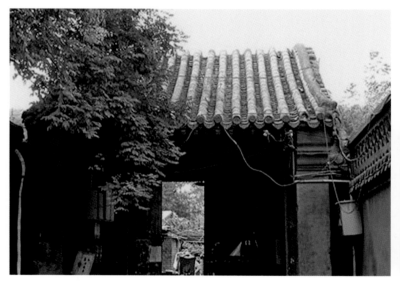

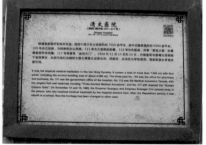

清太医院旧址

清太医院建于清光绪二十八年 (1902)，位于地安门外皇城根、兵仗局东（今北京市东城区地安门东大街 105—170 号），总占地面积 7000 余平方米。靠东边的 105 号院是三进院，是药房和日常管理办公用房。111 号院则是当年太医院的衙署，太医院办公大堂于 1968 年被大火烧毁。113 号院至 115 号院是太医院的"先医庙"。作为当时的行政主管机构，大堂设先医庙和药王庙（铜人庙）；二堂内东设"首领厅"、"庶务处"，西设"医学馆"、"教习室"。今大堂已拆建，但仍能看见当年的础石。二堂及东西厅房均保留原建筑。

刘学春提供

Site of Qing Dynasty Imperial Academy of Medicine

Founded in the 28th year under the reign of Emperor Guangxu of the Qing Dynasty, the Academy is situated closely to the city wall outside of Dian Gate and east to the old Bingzhangju (a bureau in charge of armaments in Qing's Court, now at No. 105-170, the East Street behind Dian Gate, Dongcheng District of Beijing), with an area over 7,000 square meters. The eastern Court No. 105, with three halls and two enclosed yards, once was for pharmacy and its administration. Court No. 111 was the yamen office of the Academy, but the principal hall was destroyed in a fire in 1968. Courts No. 113 to 115 were the "Temple of Ancestral Physicians". "Temple of Ancestral Physicians" and "Temple of King of Medicine" (also known as Temple of Bronze Figure) were set in the principal hall as the administrative organ, while in the secondary hall were "the Chief's Office" and "the General Affair's Office" on the east and "the Medical Library" and "the Class Room" on the west. Though disassembled, the principal hall can still be vaguely figured out with its footstones. Fortunately, the secondary hall and its east and west wings are still well preserved.

Provided by Liu Xuechun

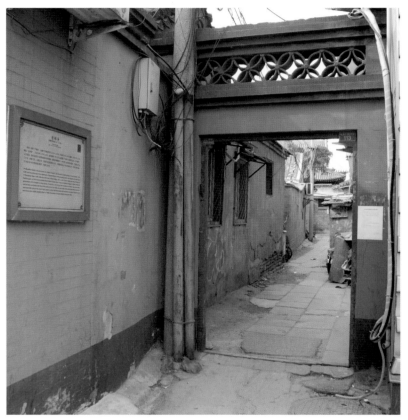

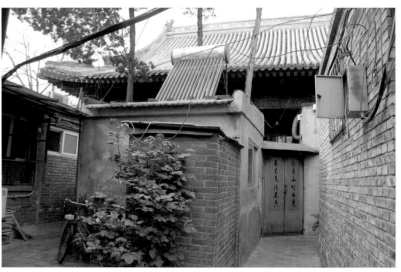

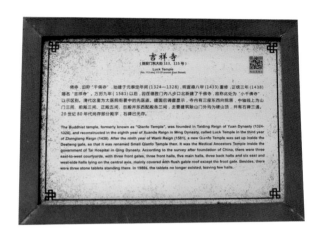

先医庙旧址

吉祥寺始建于元泰定年间（1324—1328），清光绪年间为太医院医蜀中的先医庙，位于地安门东大街 113、115 号，旧称"千佛寺"、"吉祥寺"，供奉伏羲、神农及黄帝。院内建筑错乱，百姓杂居。本图摄于 2017 年 4 月。

刘学春提供

Site of Temple of Ancestral Physicians

Temple of Good Luck, built in years under the reign of Emperor Taiding of the Yuan Dynasty (1324-1328), was renamed as "Temple of Ancestral Physicians" by the Imperial Academy of Medicine during the reign of Guangxu of the Qing Dynasty. Located at No. 113 and 115 of the East Street behind Dian Gate, it was also formerly known as "Temple of Thousand Buddhas" or "Temple of Good Luck", worshipping ancestors such as Fuxi, Shennong and the Yellow Emperor. The temple is inhabited by local residents with messy huts. The picture was taken in April 2017.
Provided by Liu Xuechun

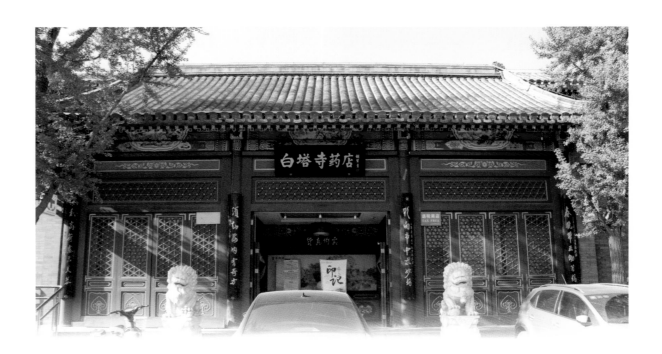

琪卉堂、大和堂旧址

1917 年，宫廷太医吴霭廷开设琪卉堂，1918 年王子丰的大和堂开业，两个药店皆位于北京市西城区阜成门内大街 165 号。1942 年，"琪卉堂"和"大和堂"先后被谢康夫买下，名称改为"北京琪卉堂新记"和"北京大和堂新记"。1953 年，两个药铺归国有。20 世纪 70 年代末在原址翻盖五层大楼，更名为"白塔寺药店"，经营面积 1200 余平方米。本图摄于 2017 年 4 月。

刘学春提供

Site of Qi Hui Tang Pharmacy and Da He Tang Pharmacy

Qi Hui Tang was founded by Wu Aiting, an imperial physician in 1917, and Da he Tang by Wang Zifeng in 1918. These two pharmacies shared the same front at No. 165, Fuchengmen Nei Street, Xicheng District of Beijing. Taken over by Xie Kangfu in 1942, they were renamed as "New Beijing Qi Hui Tang" and "New Beijing Da He Tang". In 1953, both were nationalized and run by the state. In the 1970s, they were renovated into a five-story building with an area of over 1,200 Square meters, and named as "Bai Ta Si Pharmacy". The picture was taken in April 2017.

Provided by Liu Xuechun

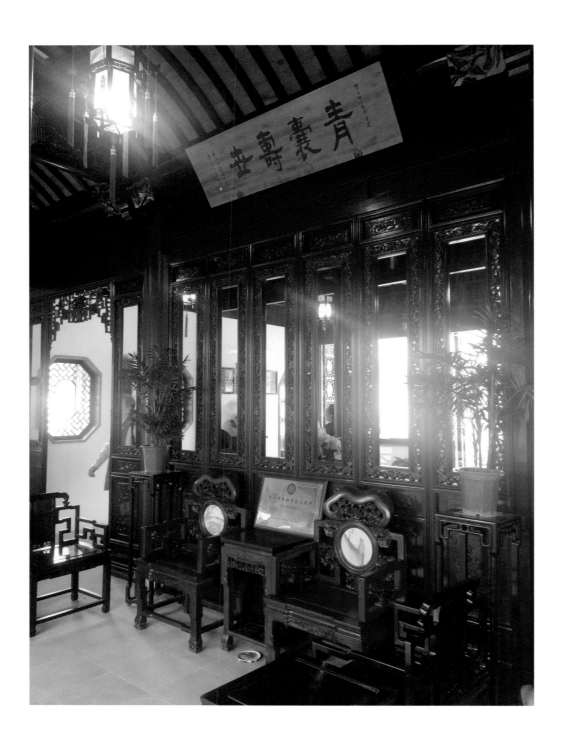

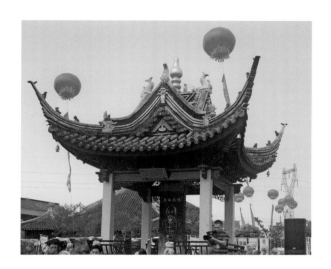

丁甘仁故居

丁甘仁故居位于江苏武进（今常州）通江乡孟河镇。丁甘仁（1866—1926）是近代伟大的中医教育先驱，上海中医专门学校创始人。1916与谢立恒、夏应堂等人创办上海中医专门学校。1921年筹建上海中医学会，亲任会长。1922年创办《中医杂志》。该图片摄于2015年秋纪念丁甘仁先生诞辰150周年活动仪式。

刘学春提供

Ding Ganren's Former Residence

Ding Ganren (1866–1926) used to live at Menghe Village, Tongjiang Town, Wujin (now known as Changzhou), Jiangsu Province. Ding was revered as a pioneer of modern TCM education, and the founder of Shanghai TCM Academy. He established the Academy with Xie Liheng and Xia Yingtang in 1916, founded Shanghai TCM Association with himself as the first commissioner in 1921, and started with *Journal of TCM* in 1922. The picture was taken in the fall of 2015 when the 150th anniversary of Ding's birth was celebrated. Provided by Liu Xuechun

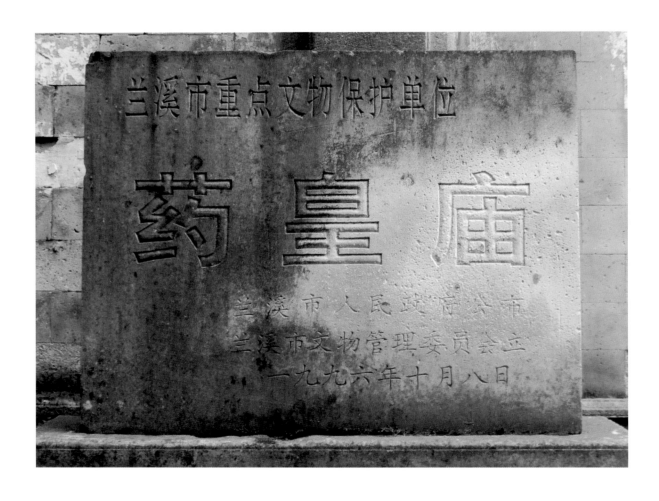

兰溪药皇庙遗址

清末民初创建的浙江省兰溪药王庙，位于雀门巷 23 号，同时也是药业公所、兰溪中医专门学校所在地。

朱德明提供

Site of Temple of King of Medicine in Lanxi

The temple, built in the late Qing Dynasty or the early Republic of China, is located at No. 23, Quemen Lane, Lanxi County City, Jinhua City in Zhejiang Province. On the site now sit both Lanxi Pharmaceutical Association and Lanxi TCM Academy.

Provided by Zhu Deming

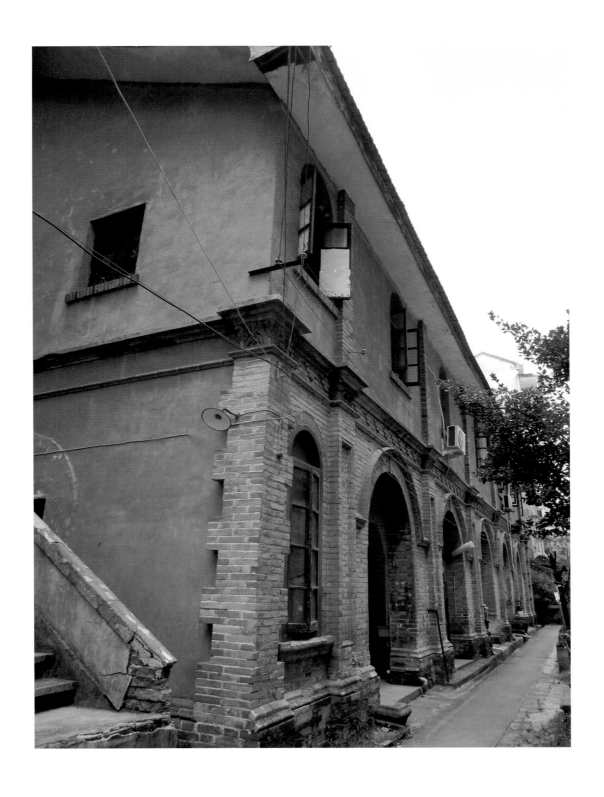

嵊州市芷湘医院遗址

1919 年 1 月，浙江省嵊县（今嵊州市）普义乡白泥墩村
王芷湘的儿子邈达、晓籁、孝本兄弟建芷湘医院，王邈达
任董事长兼院长，院址位于嵊州市城西鹿胎山南麓。

朱德明提供

Site of Zhixiang Hospital in Shengzhou City

In January 1919, Zhixiang Hospital was founded by the
Wang family (i.e. Miaoda, Xiaolai, Xiaoben, sons of Wang
Zhixiang) from Bainidun Village, Puyi Town, Sheng County
(now as Shengzhou City) in Zhejiang Province. Wang
Miaoda served as board chairman and director. The hospital
was situated at the southern foot of Lutai Mountain west to
the Shengzhou City.

Provided by Zhu Deming

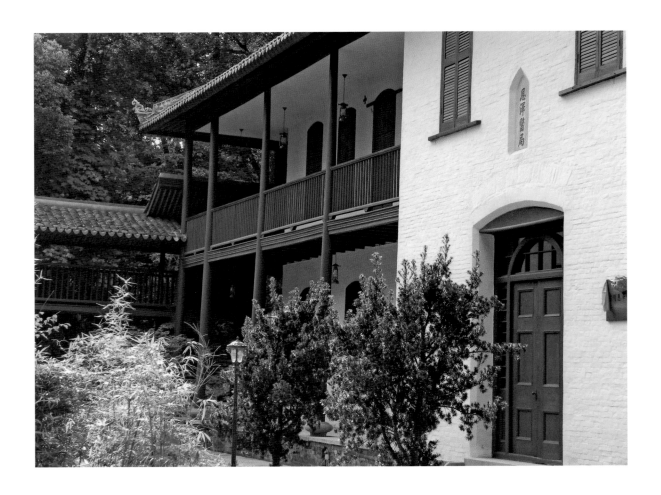

恩泽医局遗址

光绪二十七年（1901），英国传教士白明登创建恩泽医局，地处今浙江省临海市古城文化社区，现属台州学院医学院。恩泽医局由3座楼构成，北面为主楼，西侧由两座廊桥连接两幢附屋，门窗呈教堂式尖顶。

朱德明提供

Site of Enze Hospital

Enze Hospital, established in 1901 by Bai Mingdeng, a British missionary, now belongs to the Medicine School of Taizhou University. It was located on today's Ancient City Culture Community in Linhai City, Zhejiang Province. It consists of three buildings, among which the north part is the main building and the west part has two outhouses connected by two lounge bridges, with their windows and doors in the shape of church spires.

Provided by Zhu Deming

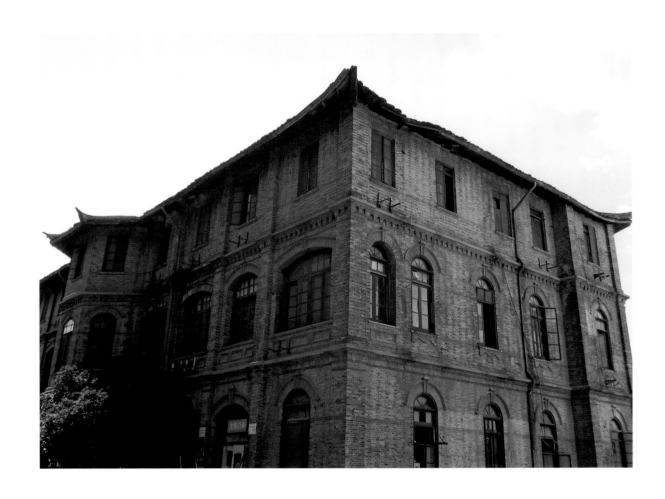

福康医院遗址

1907 年初，美国基督教北美浸礼会国外宣道会高福林在浙江省绍兴购得地皮，1907 年 3 月动工建造医院，1910 年 3 月 10 日竣工。1912 年 2 月 23 日，福康医院正式开张，这是中国境内第一家西医医院，院址绍兴南街马坊桥（今延安路）。

朱德明提供

Site of Fukang Hospital

In early 1907, Gao Fulin, a missionary of American Baptist Church, launched the construction of Fukang Hospital on a piece of purchased land in Shaoxing, Zhejiang. Completed on March 10, 1910, the hospital was formally opened on February 23, 1912. Fukang, located at Mafang Bridge, South Street (now as Yan'an Road) of Shaoxing, was the first hospital of western medicine in China.

Provided by Zhu Deming

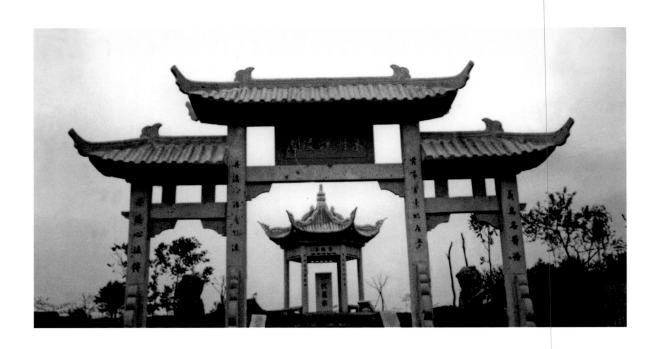

朱丹溪陵园

陵园位于浙江省义乌市赤岸镇东朱村，是元代名医朱丹溪之墓，1992 年建园。园林内有陈敏章题写的"一代宗医"石碑。朱丹溪（1281—1358），名震亨，浙江义乌市赤岸人，倡导滋阴学说，创立丹溪字派，与刘完素、张从正、李东垣一起，誉为"金元四大医家"。其著有《格致余论》《局方发挥》《本草衍义补遗》《伤寒论辨》《外科精要发挥》等。此图为 1993 年摄于修建后的义乌朱丹溪陵园正门。

Zhu Danxi's Cemetery

Zhu Danxi's tomb is at Dongzhu Village, Chi'an Town, Yiwu County, Zhejiang Province. It was restored into a cemetery in 1992. In the cemetery stands a gravestone with an inscription of "Master Physician" by late Minister of Health Chen Minzhang. Zhu Danxi (1281–1358), born locally in Chi'an, was an advocator of Nourishing Yin Therapy. As the founder of Danxi School, he was reputed as one of "the Four Great Physicians in the Jin and Yuan Dynasties" (together with Liu Wansu, Zhang Congzheng, Li Dongyuan). His classic works are "Ge Zhi Yu Lun" (*Extended Metaphysical Medicine*), "Ju Fang Fa Hui" (*Elaboration of Dispensary Formulas*), "Ben Cao Yan Yi Bu Yi" (*Addenda to Augmented Illustration on Materia Medica*), "Shang Han Lun Bian" (*Treatise on Febrile Diseases*), and "Wai Ke Jing Yao Fa Hui" (*Elaboration of Essentials of External Diseases*). This picture, taken in 1993, shows the renewed front gate.

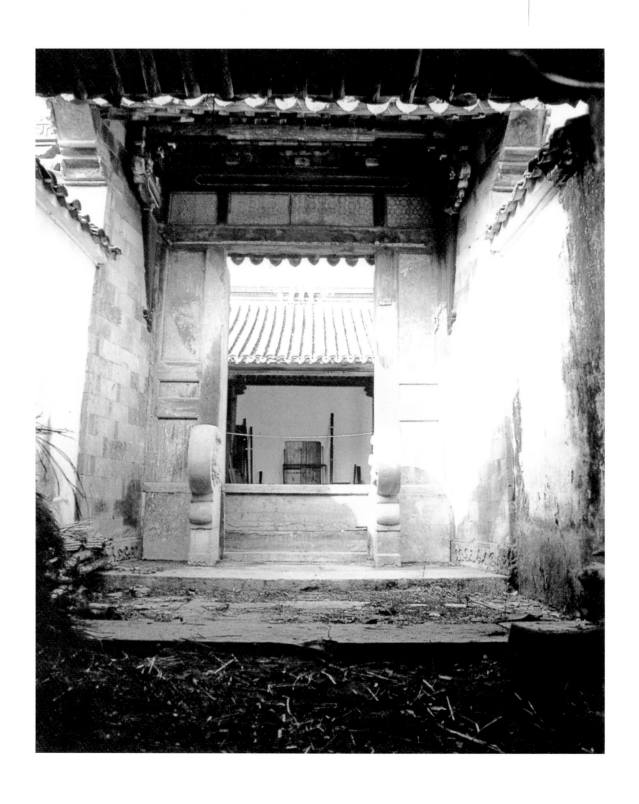

吴有性故居——凝德堂

吴有性，明末著名医学家，著《温疫论》一书创论外感瘟疫病因及传播途径，开我国传染病学之先河。其故居凝德堂位于江苏省苏州市东山镇殿新村，原堂规模较大，今仅存门厅和内厅，建筑彩绘艺术堪称明代民间苏式之典型。1981 年江苏省政府曾拨专款修葺。

Ning De Hall, Former Residence of Wu Youxing

Wu Youxing was a famous medical scientist in late Ming Dynasty. His book "Wen Yi Lun" discusses the causes and ways of plague. It started infectious disease study in China. Ningde Hall, his former residence, is located in Dianxin Village, Dongshan Town, Suzhou City, Jiangsu Province, and its architectural colour painting is typical of Suzhou folk style in the Ming Dynasty. The original hall had a large scale; however, today only a foyer and an indoor hall can be seen. In 1981, Jiangsu provincial government had allotted money for its renovation.

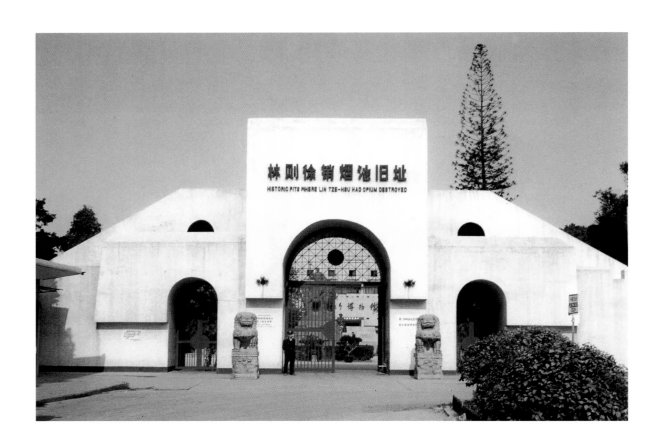

林则徐销烟池旧址门景

其位于今广东省东莞市虎门镇。19 世纪 30
年代英国、葡萄牙等武装鸦片走私到我国南
方边陲，危害我国人民健康。林则徐虎门销
烟查办鸦片 2 万多箱。1839 年 6 月 3 日，
林则徐下令在虎门销烟地当众销毁鸦片。此
为整修后照片。

Lin Zexu's Opium Combustion Pit

The Opium Combustion Pit is sited in Humen
Town, Dongguan City, Guangdong Province.
In the 1830s a gang of English and Portuguese
armed smugglers shipped and dumped opium
in Chinese southern border areas. The opium
turned out to be extraordinarily detrimental to
Chinese civilians' health. Lin Zexu, Viceroy of
Guangdong and Guangxi and Imperial Envoy of
Emperor Daoguang, forcefully impounded over
20,000 chests of opium. On June 3, 1839, Lin
ordered to destroy the opium publicly in a lime pit
in Humen. The picture shows the renewed pit.

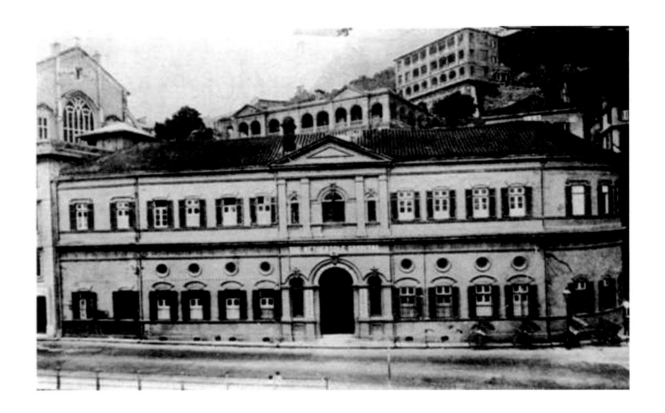

香港那打素医院

香港于 1887 年建雅丽氏医院，于 1893 年建那打素医院，于 1906 年建何妙龄医院，先后作为香港西医书院的教学医院，今已合并为香港雅丽氏何妙龄那打素医院，一般称为那打素医院。该院位于港岛般咸道，由中华基督教会管理，并曾由港英政府医管局资助开支。

Hong Kong Nethersole Hospital

Hong Kong established Alice Memorial Hospital in 1887, Nethersole Hospital in 1893 and Ho Miu Ling Hospital in 1906, all of which successively served as the teaching hospitals of the College of Medicine. At present, they are combined into the Alice Ho Miu Ling Nethersole Hospital which is generally called Nethersole Hospital. Located in Bonham Road, it is governed by the Chinese Christian Church and the Health Authority of the British Hong Kong Government once aided the hospital financially.

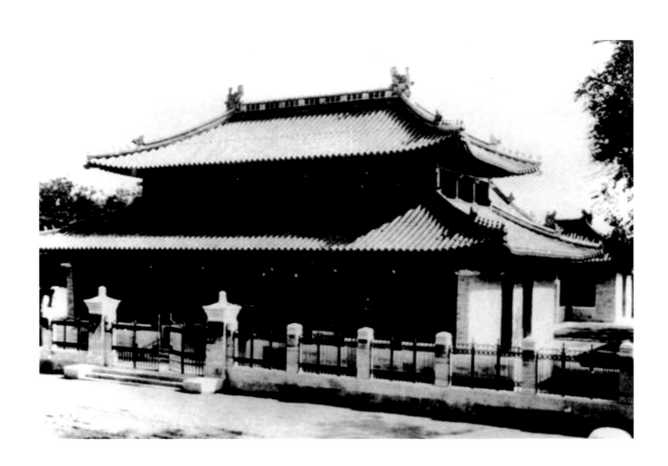

北京协和医学堂

1906 年英、美教会在北京合办协和医学堂，1915 年美国洛克菲勒基金会医药部将其接管并扩充为北京协和医学院，成为当时国内最大的教会医学院。其后北京协和医学院曾数次改名，今称中国医学科学院北京协和医学院。图为 1925 年建成使用的图书馆楼。

Peking Union Medical College

In 1906, British and American churches jointly founded the Union Medical College in Beijing. Then in 1915, the Medical Department of the Rockefeller Foundation took charge of it and expanded it into Peking Union Medical College, which became the largest church school of medicine in China at that time. After several times of name changing, it is now called Chinese Academy of Medical Sciences & Peking Union Medical College. The picture shows the library building completed in 1925.

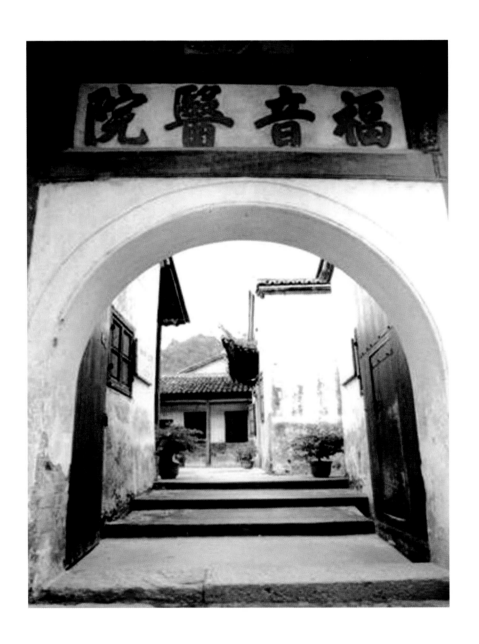

福音医院原址

英国伦敦公会在福建汀州（位于今福建长汀县）创办福音医院。1925 年傅连暲接任院长。1927 年 8 月该院收治南昌起义伤病员 300 余人。1933 年，傅连暲将医院全部设备迁往瑞金，建立中央红色医院。

Former Site of Evangelismos Hospital

This hospital was founded by the London Guild in Tingzhou, Fujian Province. In 1925, Fu Lianzhang became the director of this hospital. In August 1927, this hospital received and cured more than 300 wounded patients in Nanchang Uprising. In 1933, Fu Lianzhang moved all the equipments of this hospital to Ruijin, Jiangxi Province where he established the Central Red Hospital.

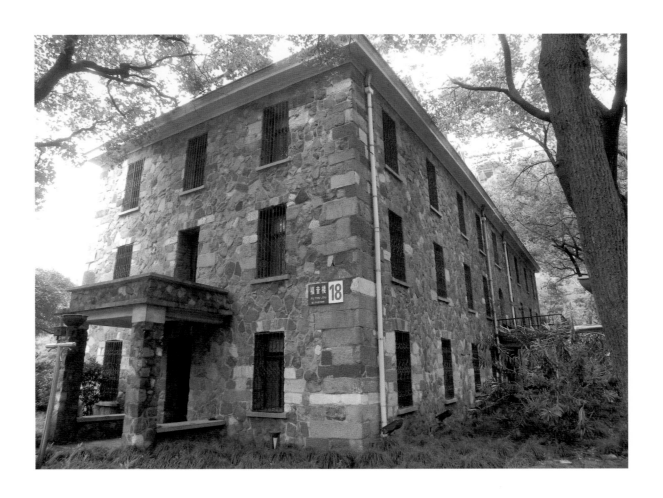

福音医院福音楼遗址

湖州吴兴福音医院建于 1912 年，是由美国在华传教的基督教监理会办的湖郡医院和中华基督教浸礼会公会办的福音医院于 1915 年秋合并而成。该院初创时租赁马军巷吴济清的 5 间房屋（今马军巷 213 号），孟杰任首任院长。

朱德明提供

Site of Gospel Building in Gospel Hospital

Founded in 1912, Gospel Hospital (in Wuxing district, Huzhou city) was later merged by Hujun Hospital which was founded by the American Christian Supervisory Commission that did missionary work in China and Gospel Hospital which was founded by China Baptist Guild in autumn, 1915. At the initial stage it rented five rooms of Wu Jiqing at Majun Alley, which is now at No. 213 Majun Alley. And Meng Jie was the first director of this hospital.

Provided by Zhu Deming

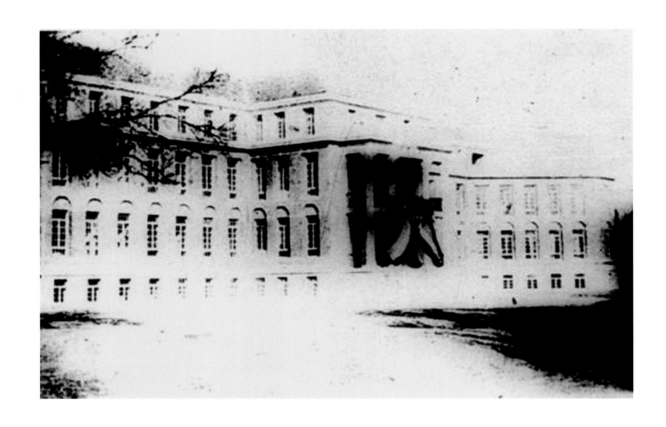

北京中央医院外景

北京中央医院 1918 年创办，系第一所中国人集资建立的西医医院，由伍连德创建，位于今北京大学人民医院所在地。

Exterior Scene of Beijing Central Hospital

Beijing Central Hospital, established in 1918 by Wu lien-teh, was the first western medicine hospital founded by Chinese people. It was located on present site of the People's Hospital of Beijing Medical University.

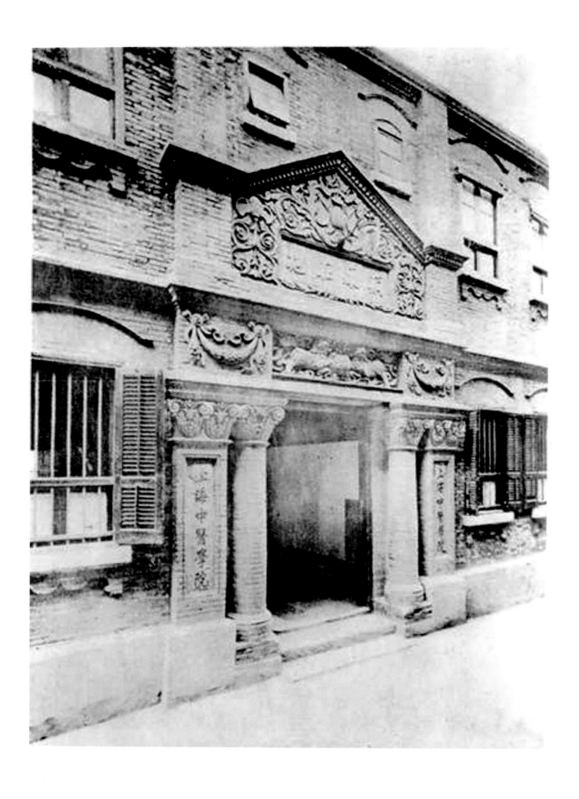

上海中医药大学民国时期院址

上海中医药大学前身是丁甘仁等创办的上海中医专门学校，创立于 1917 年。首任校长谢观。1931 年其改名为上海中医学院。早期教师有曹颖甫、丁福保、陆渊雷、祝味菊等，毕业生丁济万、陈存仁、秦伯未、章次公、程门雪、黄文东等后皆成为近现代名医。

Site of Shanghai University of Traditional Chinese Medicine in the Period of the Republic of China

Shanghai University of Traditional Chinese Medicine, renamed in 1931, grew out of the Shanghai Specialised School of Traditional Chinese Medicine, which was founded in 1917 by Ding Ganren and other people, with Xie Guan as its first principal. The early teachers include Cao Yingfu, Ding Fubao, Lu Yuanlei and Zhu Weiju, etc. And the early graduates, such as Ding Jiwan, Chen Cunren, Qin Bowei, Zhang Cigong, Cheng Menxue and Huang Wendong, later became famous doctors in modern China.

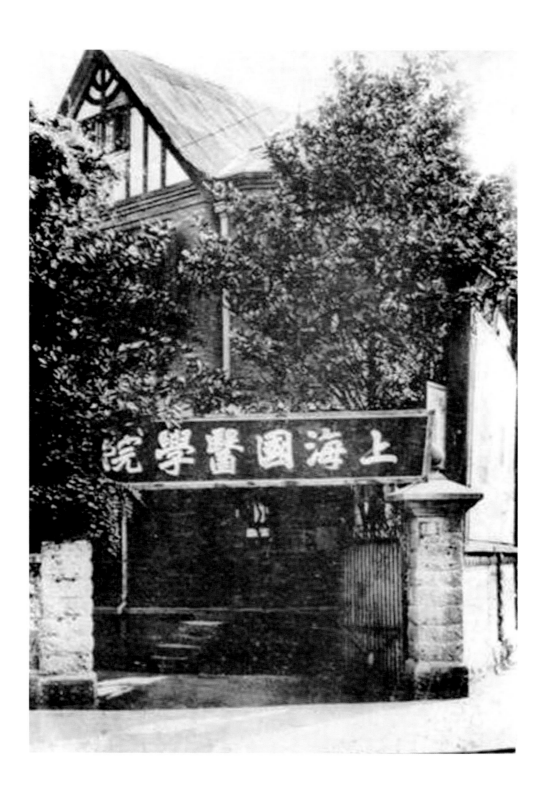

上海国医学院院址

上海国医学院 1929 年春成立。章太炎任院长，陆渊雷、章次公、徐衡之等任教，以"发煌古义，融会新知"为院训。

Site of Shanghai National Medical College

In the spring of 1929, Shanghai National Medical College was established, with Zhang Taiyan as its first president, Lu Yuanlei, Zhang Cigong and Xu Hengzhi and others as professors. The motto of this college was "Attaching importance to classics and absorbing new knowledge".

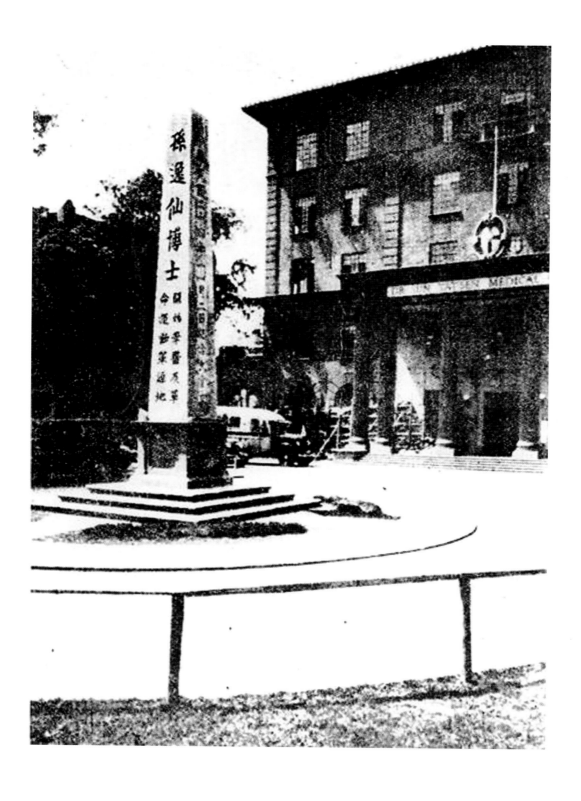

孙中山学医及革命活动纪念碑

此"孙逸仙博士开始学医及革命运动策源地"纪念碑，1935 年建，位于今广州市中山大学孙逸仙纪念医院（中山大学附属第二医院）门前。

Monument to Sun Yat-sen's Medicine Study and Revolutionary Activities

The monument was built in 1935. On the front of the monument is an inscription, which reads "The place where Dr. Sun Yat-sen began his medicine study and started his revolutionary activities". It is located in front of Sun Yat-sen Memorial Hospital, Sun Yat-sen University (the Second Affiliated Hospital of Sun Yat-sen University) in Guangzhou.

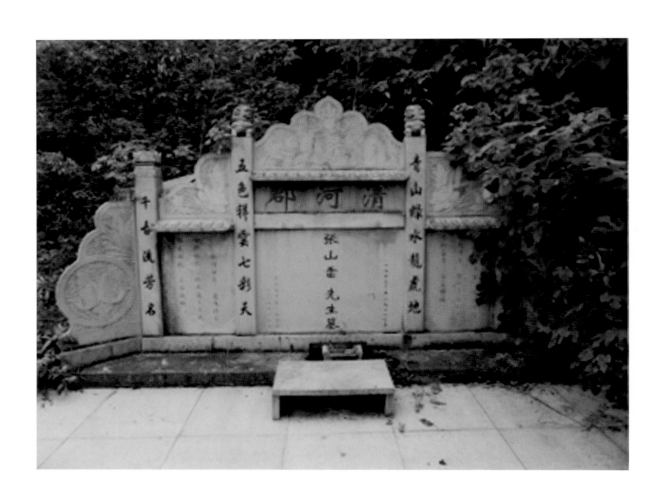

张山雷墓

张山雷（1873—1934），1920 年夏，由上海神州医学会介绍，应浙江兰溪中医专门学校之聘，任教务主任。其擅长内、妇科，对外科证治亦别具卓见。他在兰溪任教 15 年，受业学生达 600 多人，遍布江、浙、皖、赣、沪等省市。

朱德明提供

Zhang Shanlei's Tomb

Zhang Shanlei (1873–1934) was a medical specialist. In the summer 1920 on the recommendation of Shenzhou Medical Association in Shanghai, he was employed as the teaching director by Lanxi TCM Academy in Zhejiang. Zhang was expert in internal medicine and gynaecology, and also proficient in surgery diagnosis. Having taught for 15 years in Lanxi, he instructed as many as 600 students, most of whom worked in the east provinces of Jiangsu, Zhejiang, Anhui, Jiangxi and Shanghai of China.

Provided by Zhu Deming

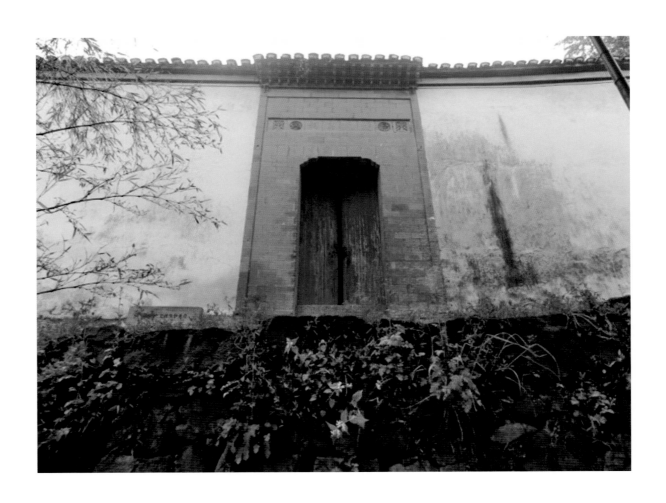

新四军苏浙军区十六旅后方医院

民国三十二年（1943）夏，新四军苏浙军区
十六旅后方医院、疗养所，迁到浙江省长兴
县白岘乡三州山村茅山自然村施家祠堂，院
长马慧明。

朱德明提供

Site of the Base Hospital and Nursing Home of Brigade 16, Jiangsu-Zhejiang Region of the New Fourth Army

In the summer of the 32nd year of Republic of
China (1943), Brigade 16, Jiangsu-Zhejiang
Region of the New Fourth Army transferred
its base hospital and nursing home to Shi's
Ancestral Hall at Maoshan Village, Baixian
Town, Changxing County in Zhejiang Province.
Ma Huiming directed the hospital at that time.
Provided by Zhu Deming

索　引

（所在地按拼音字母排序）

Index

参考文献

[1] 李经纬. 中国古代医史图录 [M]. 北京：人民卫生出版社，1992.

[2] 傅维康，李经纬，林昭庚. 中国医学通史：文物图谱卷 [M]. 北京：人民卫生出版社，2000.

[3] 和中浚，吴鸿洲. 中华医学文物图集 [M]. 成都：四川人民出版社，2001.

[4] 上海中医药博物馆. 上海中医药博物馆馆藏珍品 [M]. 上海：上海科学技术出版社，2013.

[5] 西藏自治区博物馆. 西藏博物馆 [M]. 北京：五洲传播出版社，2005.

[6] 崔乐泉. 中国古代体育文物图录：中英文本 [M]. 北京：中华书局，2000.

[7] 张金明，陆雪春. 中国古铜镜鉴赏图录 [M]. 北京：中国民族摄影艺术出版社，2002.

[8] 文物精华编辑委员会. 文物精华 [M]. 北京：文物出版社，1964.

[9] 谭维四. 湖北出土文物精华 [M]. 武汉：湖北教育出版社，2001.

[10] 常州市博物馆. 常州文物精华 [M]. 北京：文物出版社，1998.

[11] 镇江博物馆. 镇江文物精华 [M]. 合肥：黄山书社，1997.

[12] 贵州省文化厅，贵州省博物馆. 贵州文物精华 [M]. 贵阳：贵州人民出版社，2005.

[13] 徐良玉. 扬州馆藏文物精华 [M]. 南京：江苏古籍出版社，2001.

[14] 昭陵博物馆，陕西历史博物馆. 昭陵文物精华 [M]. 西安：陕西人民美术出版社，1991.

[15] 南通博物苑. 南通博物苑文物精华 [M]. 北京：文物出版社，2005.

[16] 邯郸市文物研究所. 邯郸文物精华 [M]. 北京：文物出版社，2005.

[17] 张秀生，刘友恒，聂连顺，等. 中国河北正定文物精华 [M]. 北京：文化艺术出版社，1998.

[18] 陕西省咸阳市文物局. 咸阳文物精华 [M]. 北京：文物出版社，2002.

[19] 安阳市文物管理局. 安阳文物精华 [M]. 北京：文物出版社，2004.

[20] 深圳市博物馆. 深圳市博物馆文物精华 [M]. 北京：文物出版社，1998.

[21]《中国文物精华》编辑委员会. 中国文物精华（1993）[M]. 北京：文物出版社，1993.

[22] 夏路，刘永生．山西省博物馆馆藏文物精华 [M]. 太原：山西人民出版社，1999.

[23] 文物精华编辑委员会．文物精华 [M]. 北京：文物出版社，1957.

[24] 山西博物院，湖北省博物馆．荆楚长歌：九连墩楚墓出土文物精华 [M]. 太原：山西人民出版社，2011.

[25] 刘广堂，石金鸣，宋建忠．晋国雄风：山西出土两周文物精华 [M]. 沈阳：万卷出版公司，2009.

[26] 沈君山，王国平，单迎红．滦平博物馆馆藏文物精华 [M]. 北京：中国文联出版社，2012.

[27] 张家口市博物馆．张家口市博物馆馆藏文物精华 [M]. 北京：科学出版社，2011.

[28] 浙江省文物考古研究所．浙江考古精华 [M]. 北京：文物出版社，1999.

[29] 故宫博物院．故宫雕刻珍萃 [M]. 北京：紫禁城出版社，2004.

[30] 故宫博物院紫禁城出版社．故宫博物院藏宝录 [M]. 上海：上海文艺出版社，1986.

[31] 首都博物馆．大元三都 [M]. 北京：科学出版社，2016.

[32] 新疆维吾尔自治区博物馆．新疆出土文物 [M]. 北京：文物出版社，1975.

[33] 王兴伊，段逸山．新疆出土涉医文书辑校 [M]. 上海：上海科学技术出版社，2016.

[34] 刘学春．刍议医药卫生文物的概念与分类标准 [J]. 中华中医药杂志，2016，31（11）:4406-4409.

[35] 上海古籍出版社．中国艺海 [M]. 上海：上海古籍出版社，1994.

[36] 紫都，岳鑫．一生必知的 200 件国宝 [M]. 呼和浩特：远方出版社，2005.

[37] 谭维四．湖北出土文物精华 [M]. 武汉：湖北教育出版社，2001.

[38] 张建青．青海彩陶收藏与鉴赏 [M]. 北京：中国文史出版社，2007.

[39] 银景琦．仡佬族文物 [M]. 南宁：广西人民出版社，2014.

[40] 廖果，梁峻，李经纬．东西方医学的反思与前瞻 [M]. 北京：中医古籍出版社，2002.

[41] 梁峻，张志斌，廖果，等．中华医药文明史集论 [M]. 北京：中医古籍出版社，2003.

[42] 郑蓉，庄乾竹，刘聪，等．中国医药文化遗产考论 [M]. 北京：中医古籍出版社，2005.